Recollecting Freud

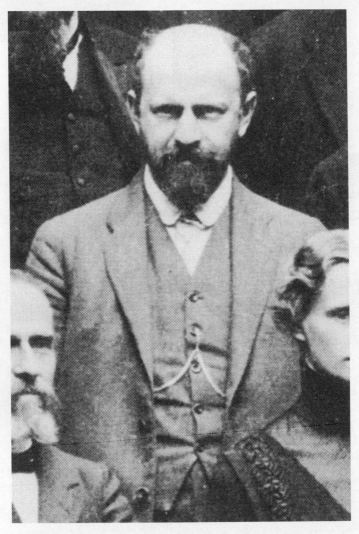

Isidor Sadger as he appeared at the 1911 Weimar Congress

Recollecting Freud

Isidor Sadger

Edited by
Alan Dundes

Translated by
Johanna Micaela Jacobsen
and
Alan Dundes

The University of Wisconsin Press

The University of Wisconsin Press
1930 Monroe Street, 3rd Floor
Madison, Wisconsin 53711-2059
uwpress.wisc.edu

3 Henrietta Street
London WC2E 8LU, England
eurospanbookstore.com

Printed in the United States of America

Library of Congress Cataloging-in-Publication Data
Sadger, J.
[Sigmund Freud. English]
Recollecting Freud / Isidor Sadger; edited by Alan Dundes;
translated by Johanna Micaela Jacobsen and Alan Dundes.
p.   cm.
ISBN 0-299-21100-2 (hardcover: alk. paper)
1. Freud, Sigmund, 1856–1939.
2. Psychoanalysts—Austria—Biography.
I. Dundes, Alan.   II. Title.
BF109.F74S2413   2005
150.19′52′092—dc22′   2004025672

ISBN 978-0-299-21104-2 (pbk.: alk. paper)
ISBN 978-0-299-21103-5 (e-book)

Contents

Introduction

Sigmund Freud, who was born on May 6, 1856, in the small town of Freiberg in what was then Moravia and who died in London on September 23, 1939, shortly after having been forced to flee from the Nazi occupation of his beloved Vienna, was without doubt one of the major figures of the twentieth century. As anyone with the slightest interest in Freud or the branch of psychiatry known as psychoanalysis can attest, there is a veritable Freud industry consisting of countless dozens of books and articles devoted to his life and work. Almost every conceivable aspect of his biography and his writings has been subjected to the most intense scrutiny and analysis, even psychoanalysis. The range of writing runs the gamut from hagiographic glorification to the most extreme Freud-bashing.

The avalanche of the Freudian literature is so great that it is doubtful whether any one individual has read every single word on the subject. The initial biographies and reminiscences were often written by those who knew him personally. Some were colleagues; others were former patients. Among the most respected sources is that written by Ernest Jones (1879–1958), one of Freud's most loyal disciples. Jones wrote a three-volume opus, *The Life and Work of Sigmund Freud* (1953, 1955, 1957). Although somewhat partisan, bordering on hagiography, Jones's admirable fifteen hundred pages of detail is probably unmatched at least in terms of overall coverage of Freud's life. Freud himself wrote a short essay entitled "An Autobiographical Study," first published in 1925, and supplemented by a "Postscript" in 1935. Among the myriad contemporary biographies of Freud, historian Peter Gay's 810-page *Freud: A Life for Our Time* (1988) is perhaps the most comprehensive, although there are many, many others, such as Ronald W. Clark's *Freud, the Man and the Cause: A Biography* (1980).

There are at least as many, if not more, books criticizing Freud as there are admiring or objective biographies. Representative (and rather telling) titles include: Marie Balmary, *Psychoanalyzing Psychoanalysis* (1982); E. M. Thornton, *The Freudian Fallacy* (1984); E. Fuller Torrey, *Freudian Fraud* (1992); Richard Webster, *Why Freud Was Wrong* (1995); and Edward Dolnick, *Madness on the Couch* (1998). For a sampling of such critics, one has only to consult such books as Paul Robinson, *Freud and His Critics* (1993), and Frederick C. Crews, *Unauthorized Freud: Doubters Confront a Legend* (1998).

There are also numerous histories of psychoanalysis, starting with Freud's own essay plus such later surveys as Reuben Fine, *A History of Psychoanalysis* (1979); Stephen A. Mitchell and Margaret J. Black, *Freud and Beyond: A History of Modern Psychoanalytic Thought* (1995); and Joseph Schwartz, *Cassandra's Daughter: A History of Psychoanalysis* (1999).

In addition, anyone concerned with Freud or the origins of psychoanalysis has available to them a wealth of reminiscences written by former patients or analysts treated by Freud or colleagues. These include: Adolph Stern, "Some Personal Psychoanalytical Experiences with Prof. Freud" (1922); A. A. Brill, "Reflections, Reminiscences of Sigmund Freud" (1940); Roy Grinker, "Reminiscences of a Personal Contact with Freud (1940); Theodor Reik, *From Thirty Years with Freud* (1940); Max Graf, "Reminiscences of Professor Sigmund Freud" (1942); Hanns Sachs, *Freud: Master and Friend* (1944); Joseph Wortis, *Fragments of an Analysis with Freud* (1954); H[ilda] D[oolittle]'s *Tribute to Freud, by H.D.* (1956); Ludwig Binswanger, *Sigmund Freud: Reminiscences of a Friendship* (1957); Ernest Jones, *Free Associations: Memoirs of a Psychoanalyst* (1959); Bruno Goetz, *Erinnerungen an Sigmund Freud* (1969); Edoardo Weiss, *Sigmund Freud as a Consultant: Recollections of a Pioneer in Psychoanalysis* (1970); Max Schur, *Freud: Living and Dying* (1972); John M. Dorsey, *An American Psychiatrist in Vienna, 1935–1937, and*

His Sigmund Freud (1976); Abram Kardiner, *My Analysis with Freud: Reminiscences* (1977); and Richard F. Sterba, *Reminiscences of a Viennese Psychoanalyst* (1982). There is even a memoir of remembrance by Freud's maid, Paula Fichtl (Berthelsen 1987), not to mention one written by one of his sons, Martin: *Glory Reflected: Sigmund Freud—Man and Father* (1957). A number of these glimpses of contact with Freud, or excerpts thereof, are contained in Ruitenbeek's excellent anthology, *Freud as We Knew Him* (1973). Generally speaking, many of these reminiscences tend to be as much if not more about their authors' lives as about Freud.

What is curious is that not a single one of the innumerable books and articles devoted to Freud, whether pro or con, has consulted one of the earliest considerations of Freud and his achievements, written by a definite insider, one of Freud's first students, and a longtime member of Freud's Wednesday Psychological Society, which eventually morphed into the Viennese Psychoanalytic Society. The book in question is *Sigmund Freud: Persönliche Erinnerungen,* by Dr. Isidor Sadger, and it was published by the Ernst Wengraf Verlag in Vienna in 1930. The ten short chapters of the book treat Freud as a teacher, therapist, and clinician, as well as his involvement in the various psychoanalytic congresses, his delight in wit, his attitudes towards Judaism, and his strong opinion concerning lay (non-medical) analysts, all topics treated endlessly by the hordes of Freudian critics that surfaced after 1930.

Questions that come to mind are: Who was Isidor Sadger? And why was his book, very likely one of the first full-fledged major considerations of Freud and his influence, totally ignored by every single scholar to date who has written about Freud?

According to Elke Mühlleitner's authoritative *Biographisches Lexikon der Psychoanalyse* (1992), which includes some one hundred fifty brief capsule biographies of the members of the Wednesday Psychological Society and the Viennese Psychoanalytic Society from 1902 to 1938, Isidor Isaak Sadger was born on October 29, 1867, in Neusandec in Galicia of Jewish parents Miriam and Hersch Sadger. He completed his medical training at the University of Vienna in 1891 and began his practice in 1893, eventually specializing in neurology. Sadger was an advocate of a treatment known as hydrotherapy, a popular procedure involving immersion in water developed in the nineteenth century by a Silesian farmer, Vincent Priessnitz (1801–1851), who had popularized the medicinal value of the external application of water as a curative technique. This "water cure" practice survives in modern times in the form of whirlpool paths and hot-tubs as well as at spas. (Consider all the German place names ending with "baden," as in Baden-Baden or Wiesbaden.) Sadger wrote several papers on hydropathy in 1896 (1896a, 1896b; May 1999: 28), and in an 1897 article Sadger proclaimed hydrotherapy as "the cure of the future" for nervous diseases (Rose 1998:70).

It was in the winter semester of 1895–96 that Sadger began to audit Freud's lectures at the University of Vienna. He continued to do so in 1896, 1898, and 1903–4. But it was his eventual participation in the Vienna Psychoanalytic Society that was the critical turning point in his involvement with Freud.

Vienna at the end of the nineteenth century and the beginning of the twentieth century was one of the most exciting intellectual centers in the world. It was not just a question of art, literature, and politics, but it was also the newly emerging branch of psychiatry known as psychoanalysis (Schorske 1980; Rose 1998; Pouh 2000). According to Wilhelm Stekel (1868–1940) in his *Autobiography,* it was he who first proposed to Freud in 1902 the idea of getting together informally. Freud liked the idea and sent postcard invitations to four individuals: Stekel, Max Kahane (1866–1928), who left the group in 1907, Rudolf Reitler (1865–1917), supposedly the first to practice psychoanalysis after Freud, and Alfred Adler (1870–1937). "I gave him the suggestion of founding a little discussion group; he accepted the idea, and every Wednesday evening after supper we met in Freud's home. . . . These first evenings were inspiring. We found some random themes to talk about and everybody participated in a real discussion. On the first night we spoke about the psychological implications of smoking. There was complete harmony among the five, no dissonances; we were like pioneers in a newly discovered land, and Freud was the leader. A spark seemed to jump from one mind to the other, and every evening was like a revelation. We were so enthralled by these meetings that we decided new members could be added to our circle only by unanimous consent. The new ones came: Paul Federn [1871–1950] and Edward Hitschmann [1871–1957], later Isidor Sadger who introduced Fritz Wittels [1880–1950]" (Stekel 1950:115–116). Apparently, the order of discussants was determined by drawing from a Greek urn slips of paper upon which those in attendance had written their names. After the drawing, members were expected to remain until the end of the meeting (Rose 1998:56–57).

Others have described the stimulating atmosphere that permeated the initial meetings of the group called the Wednesday Psychological Society. Here is the description of the remarkable ambience of the gatherings written by Max Graf (1873–1958): "We would gather in Freud's office every Wednesday evening. Freud sat at the head of a long table, listening, taking part in the discussion, smoking his cigar, and weighing every word with a serious, probing look. . . . The gatherings followed a definite ritual. First, one of the members would present a paper. Then, black coffee and cakes were served; cigars and cigarettes were on the table and were consumed in great quantities. After a social quarter of an hour, the discussion would begin. The last and the decisive word was always spoken by Freud himself. There was an atmosphere of the foundation of a religion in that room. Freud himself was its new prophet who made the theretofore prevailing methods of psychological investigation appear superficial. Freud's pupils—all inspired and convinced were his apostles. Despite the fact that the contrast among the personalities of this circle of pupils was great, at that early period of Freudian investigation all of them were united in their respect for and inspiration with Freud" (1942:470–471; for another account see Wittels 1924:133–134). There is little question that this lively group sparked an important intellectual paradigm shift in psychiatry (Gross 1979).

On April 15, 1908, the group decided to become more formalized and on October 12, 1910, finally changed its name to the Vienna Psychoanalytic Society (Jones 1955:9). It continued to exist until 1938 when the incursion of the Nazis forced its dissolution (Reichmayr 1995:179).

It was at the meeting of November 14, 1906, that Freud proposed Sadger for membership and it is noteworthy that it was Freud himself who nominated Sadger. One week later the minutes for the meeting of November 21 indicate that he was duly admitted "by unanimous vote" (Nunberg and Federn 1962:52). Sadger was notified of his acceptance the following day, Thursday, November 22.

Freud's first contact with Sadger occurred much earlier. In 1894 and 1895 Sadger wrote a series of articles on Ibsen for *Allgemeine Zeitung,* a local newspaper (May 1999:47), and in 1897 Sadger published an essay praising the writings of the well-known neurologist and psychiatrist Paul Flechsig (1847–1929), which he sent to Freud. Flechsig had treated Daniel Paul Screber (1842–1911), a famous patient whose 1903 autobiographical description of his mental state provided the data base for Freud's classic 1911 paper "Psycho-Analytic Notes upon an Autobiographical Account of a Case of Paranoia (Dementia Paranoides)" (Niederland 1974). Sadger praised Flechsig to the skies, which annoyed Freud to the point that he had a dream about it. How do we know this? We know this because Freud, as part of his remarkable self-analysis, included the dream in his ground-breaking *The Interpretation of Dreams,* first published in 1900.

Here is the dream as reported by Freud: "A colleague sent an essay of his, in which he had, in my opinion, overestimated the value of a recent physiological discovery, and had expressed himself, moreover, in extravagant terms. On the following night I dreamed a sentence which obviously referred to this essay: 'That is a truly *norekdal* style.' The solution of this word-formation at first gave me some difficulty; it was unquestionably formed as a parody of the superlatives 'colossal' 'pyramidal'; but it was not easy to say where it came from. At last the monster fell apart into the two names *Nora* and *Ekdal,* from two well-known plays by

Ibsen [*A Doll's House* and *The Wild Duck*]. I had previously read a newspaper article on Ibsen by the writer whose latest work I was now criticizing in my dream" (1938:331). Sadger is not named, and this has unfortunately led to the "colleague" being mistakenly identified as Wilhelm Fliess (1858–1928) (Anthi 1990), with whom Freud had an important intense friendship that resulted in a historically significant correspondence (Masson 1985). However, several writers have correctly identified Sadger as the colleague in question (Wittels 1924:76; May 1999, 2003). The point in the present context is that by 1900 Freud already considered Sadger a colleague, and that he had already been put off by Sadger's style of presentation.

On November 28, 1906, just one week after having been accepted into the Society, Sadger presented the first of what would prove to be his many communications to the group. In fact, with the possible exception of Freud himself, it seems that no member of the Society made more presentations than did Sadger. Entitled "Lenau and Sophie Löwenthal," the debut paper (Sadger 1909a) concerned Austrian writer Nikolaus Lenau (1802–1850), who eventually died in a mental institution. The paper reflected two of Sadger's principal research interests. Sadger was inclined to present psychological (or psychoanalytic) profiles of authors in what he termed "pathographies"—he wrote an essay about this type of analysis in *Imago* in 1912. Sadger did not invent the term pathography. In the mid-nineteenth century the term referred simply to the history or description of a disease. But as employed by Sadger (and also by Freud in his study of Da Vinci), it referred to a psychiatric study of an author or artist based upon an analysis of that individual's creative oeuvre. Sadger also had a great interest in the study of homosexuality. In his initial presentation, he suggested that Lenau's neurosis might have had a hereditary component and he also remarked that part of Lenau's personality profile included a homosexual tendency which he traced to an experience he had had at age fourteen with an unmarried cleric. Sadger further noted that "In the course of Lenau's insanity, homosexual tendencies also became manifest. He took a liking to the gardener's helper, to stable boys, and the like" (Nunberg and Federn 1962: 65). Freud's criticism on this occasion was relatively mild. He did, however, peremptorily dismiss Sadger's notion of a "hereditary neurosis." "The term 'hereditary neurosis' which the speaker used, should preferably be avoided, since it does not convey the essential character of any definite symptom complex" (65).

Sadger proposed the term again, along with "hereditary psychosis," during a discussion of "Degeneration" at a meeting on May 1, 1907, eliciting the same negative reaction from Freud. This time Freud minced no words: "The new concepts of hereditary neurosis and hereditary psychosis should be rejected" (Nunberg and

Federn 1962:185, 187). The following week, Freud reiterated his position: "Among the propositions advanced by Sadger last time . . . the diagnosis of hereditary deficiency is altogether of no value" (193). Of course, if a neurosis were truly completely hereditary, then that would eliminate the basic thesis of Freud's concept of the importance of infantile conditioning on adult personality. Adler, for example, also objected to "Sadger's theory of hereditary taint—which, according to him, is characterized by a number of qualities ('stigmata') that cannot be psychoanalytically resolved" (Nunberg and Federn 1974:76). Clearly Freud would not be at all amenable to such a concept. Sadger persisted in his use of the concept, but invariably other members of the Society objected to it as overly reductionistic and simplistic (Rose 1998:71).

On March 20, 1907, less than six months after he had been admitted to the Society, Sadger proposed his nephew Fritz Wittels for membership. Wittels was unanimously voted in one week later (Nunberg and Federn 1962:153), but his participation in the Society was intermittent, 1906 to 1910 and 1927 to 1936, compared to that of Sadger who attended meetings faithfully from 1906 to 1933 (Mühlleitner and Reichmayr 1998:1099, 1101). Interestingly enough, Wittels wrote three books (1924, 1931, 1995) about Freud. The first of these was published six years earlier than that of Sadger, but unlike Sadger, Wittels did not devote his entire book to Freud as there were individual chapters devoted to Adler, Carl Gustav Jung (1875–1961), and Stekel, a fact that surely must have displeased Freud. In contrast, Sadger's biography concentrated on Freud alone. On the other hand, we know that Freud did read Wittels's 1924 book because the English translation of it contains extracts from Freud's letter to Wittels of December 18, 1923, in which he offers comments, some critical, of Wittels's portrayal of him. In fact, Freud read the English translation too as his letter of August 15, 1924, attests, one line of which reads "Neither would a little more truthfulness have done your biography any harm" (E. Freud 1975:352). Whereas, in contrast, there is no evidence whatsoever that Freud ever read Sadger's book. This seems odd inasmuch as the book was, after all, published in 1930 in Vienna, where Freud lived.

Although Sadger has to be considered a minor figure in the early psychoanalytic movement—most histories of psychoanalysis rarely or barely mention him, and as one student of the subject noted "Little is known about Sadger" (Rose 1998:69), a phrase that is often repeated (Nunberg and Federn 1962:xxxvi; Handlbauer 1998:38)—he was certainly among the most devoted followers of Freud. Sadger's enthusiasm for Freud is signaled by the fact that he was one of the first to write a popular account and appreciation of psychoanalysis intended for the wider medical profession. Entitled "Die

Bedeutung der psychoanalytischen Methode nach Freud," it was published in the *Centralblatt für Nervenheilkunde und Psychiatrie* in 1907.

At the first psychoanalytic congress, held in Salzburg on April 27, 1908, there were only a limited number of principal speakers: Freud, Jones, Sadger, Morton Prince (1854–1929), Franz Riklin (1878–1938), Karl Abraham (1877–1925), Stekel, Adler, and Jung. The very fact that Sadger was chosen, presumably by Freud, to be one of such an illustrious group attests to his stature at that time. According to a copy of the program reproduced in *Minutes of the Vienna Psychoanalytic Society*, Sadger's communication was entitled "Contribution to the Etiology of Psychopathia Sexualis" (Nunberg and Federn 1962:389). In Ernest Jones's report of the program, the paper title is given as "The Aetiology of Homosexuality" (1955:42), and this is more or less confirmed by Wittels who claimed that at the Salzburg congress "Sadger was able to report the first case in which a homosexual had been cured by psycho-analysis" (1924:136). The presentation was published as "Zur Ätiologie der konträren Sexualempfindung" in 1909, but was apparently based on treatment of a patient for a period of only thirteen days (Lewes 1988:62)! Already in 1908, Sadger had published several papers on homosexuality, and in one of them he asked "Is homosexuality curable?" His conclusion in part: "Freud's psychoanalytic method gives us for the first time a technique that provides a basis to cure homosexuality" (1908b:720). Sadger felt that homosexuality could be cured through psychoanalysis just as sleepwalking could (1920b). Freud, however, did not share Sadger's view that homosexuality was an "illness" that could be "cured" (Lewes 1988:28–35; Robinson 2000). In another paper, published in the *Archiv für Kriminal-Anthropologie und Kriminalistik* in 1913, Sadger asked, "What is the value of narratives and autobiographies of homosexuals?" Freud acknowledged in print his debt to Sadger's investigations of homosexuality, for example, in his famous *Three Essays on the Theory of Sexuality* (1905:135) and his analysis of Leonardo Da Vinci (1910:99n.1). Freud also credited Sadger with emphasizing the basic "bisexuality of human beings" (1908:165; 1920:157).

Another indication of Sadger's early appreciation of Freud's writings is his short essay "Analerotik und Analcharakter," which appeared in 1910. It was probably the first published reaction to Freud's brilliant 1908 paper "Character and Anal Erotism." Sadger's insights were noted by both Abraham Ernest Jones in their more extensive treatments of so-called anal erotic character. However, in a somewhat mean-spirited statement, one scholar has remarked that "Sadger seemed to have made a minor career at explicating the varieties of anal erotism from buttocks erotism *(Gesässerotik)* to urethral erotism" (Lewes 1988:58) referring to essays written in 1910 and 1913.

Sadger's admiration for Freud and his work is also demonstrated in his review of *The Interpretation of Dreams* in the folklore journal *Anthropophyteia* in 1911. His last sentence: "This book has become for all its students a classic" (1911:490). Curiously enough, Sadger's rave review contains an egregious Freudian slip. According to Kiell (1988:184) Sadger presumably meant to say: "However, Freud's genius *produced* [bringen etwas] additional priceless fruits from his work on dreams," but instead the preposition "um" was somehow inserted so that the line read "However, Freud's genius *was deprived of* [bringen um etwas] additional priceless fruits from his work on dreams." What this suggests is that by 1911, Sadger had developed some ambivalence, perhaps unconscious, in his attitude towards Freud.

To be sure, Freud's attitude towards Sadger was not altogether positive, to put it mildly. Just prior to the Salzburg congress, which took place in April 1908, Freud wrote a letter to Jung with whom he was still on very good terms. In that letter of March 5, Freud had this to say about Sadger: "I hear that Sadger, that congenital fanatic of orthodoxy, who happens by mere accident to believe in psychoanalysis rather than in the law given by God on Sinai-Horeb" (McGuire 1974:130). Freud's comment is remarkably parallel to a passage in a letter written by Abraham to Max Eitingon (1881–1943) in which Abraham tells of his experience attending a meeting of the Vienna Psychoanalytic Society. "I attended a Wednesday night meeting. He [Freud] is too advanced in relation to the others. Sadger is like a Talmudic student: He interprets and applies every rule pronounced by the master with the rigor of an orthodox Jew" (H. C. Abraham 1974:81).

The unbending rigidity of Sadger's thinking is commented upon by Richard Sterba (1898–1989) in his book of reminiscences. He recalled the reaction of some of the members of the Society to the modification of Freud's initial id-ego-superego formulation that Freud proposed in his 1923 *The Ego and the Id*. "The need to accept the new structural theory which to a great extent replaced the topographical model that until then had been the foundation of Freud's metapsychology met with great resistance. Some of the members refused to deal with it altogether. I remember that, in a theoretical discussion at a society meeting, Isidor Sadger, an older member, shouted indignantly: 'I don't care a hoot whether the id represses the ego or the ego represses the id.' He refused even to try to comprehend the change to new theoretical conceptions that Freud's *Ego and the Id* had forced upon us" (Sterba 1982:76).

Freud and other members of the Vienna Psychoanalytic Society had several objections to Sadger's various research efforts. Not only did Sadger apply Freudian theory in a rather rigid Procrustean mechanical fashion, but he did so with a kind of overkill, often presenting an undigested overwhelming mass of data. He also seemed to select relatively obscure literary figures to feature in his pathographies. In a letter to Jung dated January 2, 1910, Freud counseled him to try to rein in Sadger. "I should like to incite you to stem the interminable flow of Sadger's rubbish on the biography of *un*important men. I know the piece, like all Sadger's papers, it must to the barber's, as Hamlet says" (McGuire 1974: 283). The allusion to *Hamlet* (II, ii) is obviously a hint that Sadger's paper should be cut or at least trimmed. In another letter to Jung, dated one month later, February 2, 1910, Freud referred unhappily to the prospect of having Sadger submit a paper for the *Jahrbuch der Psychoanalyse* in no uncertain terms: "Sadger's writing is insufferable, he would only mess up our nice book" (291). On the other hand, Freud also mentioned to Jung that compared to Adler and Federn, "Sadger is the ablest practitioner" (204). Sadger may have been practicing psychoanalysis as early as 1898 (May 1999:40), and if this is so, he was one of the very first psychoanalysts. Still, on balance, Freud was beginning to find Sadger something of a trial. In a letter to Abraham dated January 14, 1912, speaking of Abraham's plan to consider Amenhotem IV in the light of psychoanalysis, Freud remarked, "It is surely a great step forward in our research." Then he added jokingly, "Do you know that you are now joined with Stekel and Sadger, the '*Bêtes noires*' of psychoanalysis against which I have always been prejudiced?" (H. C. Abraham 1974:106).

Sadger was one of the few early psychoanalysts who was not himself analyzed. This is somewhat surprising in view of the oft-repeated Freudian dictum that "The only way to learn analysis is to be psychoanalyzed" (Stern 1922:22; Wortis 1940:843; Von Urban 1958:193; Dufresne 1996:503). Sadger analyzed Hermine Hug-Helmut (1871–1924) and the maverick analyst Wilhelm Reich (1897–1957), but he was reportedly jealous of Reich insofar as Freud seemed to favor him over the older Sadger (Sharaf 1983:108). Evidently Sadger had vain hopes of being one of Freud's "favorite sons," a status he never attained. His obvious resentment of some of those "favorite sons" is a recurring theme in his book.

In another comment, this by Ludwig Jekels (1867–1954), we find a description of what happened when the Society meetings were held at a hall at the Vienna College of Physicians rather than in Freud's home. According to Jekels, personal conflicts arose in the larger venue. "There differences came to the fore which to my mind had various personal motives as their basis; above all, there was one to be the favorite son (of Freud) and to cut out others who were in favor with him. . . . Most often this happened between Stekel and Sadger, later [Viktor] Tausk [1879–1919] also entered the lists who loved to assail the two of them. This went so far that Freud asked me after one of the sessions: 'What does Tausk want from Sadger; he is indeed a serious scholar!'" (Roazen 1985:173).

Freud did have an inner circle of trusted colleagues and confidants: Abraham, Eitingon, Sándor Ferenczi (1873–1933), Jones, Otto Rank (1884–1939), and Hanns Sachs (1881–1947), to each of whom he gave a ring as a sign of their special status (Sachs 1944:153; Grosskurth 1991). Sadger was not part of this inner circle.

Most of Freud's comments about Sadger were in the form of private statements made in letters to members of his inner circle, but there were occasions when Freud criticized Sadger in public, usually following one of Sadger's numerous presentations to the Vienna Psychoanalytic Society. For example, on December 4, 1907, Sadger presented one of his pathographies, this one devoted to the Swiss poet Konrad Ferdinand Meyer (1825–1898), which would appear in monograph form the following year. Sadger emphasized two factors: heredity and Meyer's apparent unrequited love for his mother. Despite the audience's obvious sympathy for the Oedipal arguments, they found Sadger's analysis crude and a bit simplistic. The rigidity and reductionism of Sadger's presentation greatly irritated those assembled, who did not restrain their severe criticism. So vitriolic were the comments that Freud was forced to intervene to restore peace (Gay 1988:177). He urged "moderation," claiming that, "At the very least, Sadger's industry is to be commended, though it unfortunately is all too often expended on sterile topics."

Freud, however, had his own reservations about Sadger's overly dogmatic presentations, which he considered unimaginative (Jones 1955:342), and he then went on to further criticize Sadger: "This is not the correct way to write pathographies. . . . Sadger has a rigidly established way of working. That is, he uses a two-sided scheme: hereditary tainting and modern erotic psychology. All of life is then viewed in the light of this scheme. Sadger's investigation has not clarified anything for him [Freud]" (Nunberg and Federn 1962:257).

Freud was even forced to distance himself from Sadger's pathography of Meyer. In a letter dated November 5, 1909, to his lifelong friend, the Swiss Protestant pastor Reverend Oskar Pfister (1876–1956), Freud noted, "Incidentally, K. F. Meyer's mother and sister were denounced as sexual objects not by me but by Sadger" (Meng and Freud 1963:31).

On January 17, 1912, following Sadger's presentation entitled "From Hebbel's Boyhood," which was based on what would become a series of essays that eventually culminated in a book, *Friedrich Hebbel, ein psychoanalytischer Versuch* that was published later in 1920, Freud sought to explain "why Sadger consistently encounters opposition" whenever he speaks to the Society. Freud concludes: "He has too harsh a way of approaching delicate problems. Above all, however, he invariably neglects the whole superstructure and represents things as though the psychosexual factors which are at the deepest roots were the solutions that offered themselves at the start." Even when Freud praised Sadger, there was often a devastating undercutting addendum: "There is no objection to Sadger's interpretation, aside from the fact that it is incomplete" (Nunberg and Federn 1975:16, 17).

It seems that Sadger never married (Mühlleitner 1992:283). He may also have been something of a misogynist. On April 14, 1910, there was a debate among the members of the Vienna Psychoanalytic Society as to whether or not women should be admitted to the Society. Sadger was adamantly opposed (Nunberg and Federn 1967:477). Freud, however, despite the fact that he would later be criticized by feminists for his male bias and failure to understand women, argued that women should not be excluded on principle. (Sadger also differed with Freud on the issue of lay analysis. Sadger felt strongly that only physicians should practice psychoanalysis [Sadger 1927] while Freud generally favored lay analysis. This troublesome topic is treated in a fascinating chapter-length discussion in this book.)

Two weeks later, a vote was taken with twelve in favor and two opposed, presumably one of the two being Sadger (Handlbauer 1998:89). So Freud prevailed and of the approximately one hundred fifty members of the Vienna Psychoanalytic Society over the course of that Society's existence, there were 108 men and 43 women (Mühlleitner and Reichmayr 1998:1055). The percentage of women members rose from zero in the years 1902 to 1909 to nearly 46 percent in 1937 (Mühlleitner 2000:646). There were also apparently rumors that Sadger had misbehaved with women patients (Ferris 1997:214). Supposedly Reich criticized Sadger and others for using the guise of a medical examination as an excuse to touch their patients genitally (Sharaf 1983: 108), but this may be little more than idle gossip or malicious rumor.

The fact that Sadger never married, expressed misogynistic views, and seemed particularly interested in homosexuality makes it tempting to speculate about his own sexual inclinations. It is certainly the case that in most of his interventions and comments offered on presentations made by other members of the Society, Sadger somehow always managed to mention homosexuality. In one such comment, Sadger emphasized "the significance of the homosexual tendency in neurosis which he called attention to as early as in 1897 when he laid special stress on the bisexuality of every neurotic symptom," at which point Freud responded "To Sadger, one has to reply that it is not all true that every symptom, in addition to its other roots, also has to have homosexual roots" (Nunberg and Federn 1975:98). But Sadger was not the least bit discouraged or deterred by such criticisms. He never retreated from his earlier view stated on November 20, 1907, in which he offered the following observation: "the wish for the death of the spouse is rooted in homosexuality. Homosexuality altogether plays a far greater part in the causation of neurosis than is generally believed" (Nunberg and Federn 1962:243).

In his 1907 paper setting forth his exposition of the Freudian method, he observed, "Psychoanalysis can be mastered only by one who is able to trace every symptom back to the first four years of life and often even directly to the first year of life, and he must then further find linkages to a plethora of heterosexual as well as homosexual wishes." And he added further, "Above I have already explained that behind every single hysterical symptom stands concealed a homosexual wish" (1907:47, 49).

In a paper published much later, in 1929, Sadger remarked, "We know that at puberty nearly all human beings pass through a homosexual period. Boys wax enthusiastic for 'true' friendship, school-girls for girls of their 'set,' and it is by no means uncommon for such friendships with their inevitable admixture of sexuality to last throughout life" (1929:352). Sadger even goes so far as to argue that same-sex attachments are vital in adulthood because "in such a friendship important sexual cravings must in nature remain unsatisfied" and that in turn leads to sublimations in the form of art and science. "We see," he concludes, "how necessary is mental homosexuality" (353).

In one sense, Sadger's sexual preferences are really beside the point, but inasmuch as he himself was not averse to drawing psychological inferences from the biographies of the writers he treated in his various pathographies, it does not seem unfair to consider his life from a similar perspective. Certainly a goodly number of Sadger's publications concerned homosexuality and to the extent that one is justified in assuming that research topic choices may have a projective aspect, it is not unreasonable to speculate that Sadger's unmistakable longstanding professional interest in the subject had possible personal implications. But whatever Sadger's actual or latent sexual preferences might or might not have been, what is of interest at this point in time is his unusual contribution to our knowledge of Freud.

Piecing together snippets here and there from the *Minutes of the Vienna Psychoanalytic Society* and various memoirs written by participants of the period, one can glean the fact that Sadger appears to have been actively disliked by many, including Freud himself. A revealing editorial footnote in the *Minutes* reads: "Criticism was frequently severe, not only of Sadger, but of everyone in the circle. Subsequently, Sadger was subjected to even sharper criticism. He made himself disliked although his merits in respect to psychoanalysis are considerable" (Nunberg and Federn 1962:258n.3). Perhaps it was the constant criticism leveled at Sadger that accounted for his making a formal motion that "Personal invectives and attacks should immediately be suppressed by the Chairman [Freud] who shall be given the authority to do so" (300).

One apparent reason why Sadger was disliked had to do with his manner. Evidently, he was sometimes overly blunt if not coarse in his advocacy of Freud. An early report in the *Journal of Abnormal Psychology* in 1911 characterizes Sadger as being doctrinaire and inflexibly authoritarian. "His [Sadger's] work is not lacking in such dogmatic assertions as 'Every man is from his very beginning bisexual.' . . . *It is orthodoxy free from all timidity*" (Friedländer 1911:299, emphasis in original). A further discussion of Sadger's works reads, "The well-known hypothesis of Freud relative to the erotic origin of all psychopathic manifestations is presented, together with theoretic considerations, with an aggressiveness to the point of disgust, and it cannot be too strongly refuted" (299).

Listen to what Freud said on May 5, 1909, after Sadger's presentation (Sadger 1910b) on the writer Heinrich von Kleist (1777–1811). Freud's observations followed a comment by Stekel, who said that while the content of Sadger's views were certainly justified, "the *manner* in which Sadger treats the topic makes these things rather unattractive for the general public" (Nunberg and Federn 1967:221). Freud began his critical remarks by asking, "Why is it that, even though

Sadger makes assertions that must be accepted as correct, his communications feel strange to us, sometimes even offensive?" Freud tried to answer his own question. "Sadger must also be reproached for having a special predilection for the brutal. However, our task is not arbitrarily to speak new truths, but rather to show in what way they can be arrived at. A certain degree of tolerance must go hand in hand with a deeper understanding, especially of unconscious phenomena, if life is to remain at all bearable. Sadger apparently has not acquired this tolerance, or at least he is not capable of expressing it. And this lack of tolerance, which manifests itself in a moralistic pathos, is the second repellent aspect of his paper. Quite apart from these general weaknesses, this work seems to be wholly unreliable. Factual material is totally lacking, and with it evidence for a number of things. . . . Sadger's attempts at analyzing Kleist's works are also very weak" (224–225). Keep in mind that this criticism was made in Sadger's presence.

This was by no means the only occasion when Freud spoke his mind in public about Sadger's style of presentation. On January 5, 1910, following the third portion of Sadger's three-part case history, Freud confessed (in front of Sadger) that "the first presentations of Sadger's papers always leave him with a poorer impression than when they come out in print." Part of the problem, according to Freud, was the particular patients that Sadger analyzed. "The reasons for this antagonism lie for the most part in the subjects that Sadger usually has. This patient is an absolute swine." But some of the blame lay with Sadger: "Other motives for antagonism lie in the speaker himself, above all on account of the overwhelming mass of details that he presents, when he should be presenting only the results" (Nunberg and Federn 1967:379).

The fact that Freud was occasionally outspoken in his devastating criticism of Sadger must be taken into account in evaluating Sadger's possible bias in his reporting of his personal recollections of Freud. In that context, one might view the book as Sadger's one last opportunity to retaliate somewhat for all the verbal abuse he may have felt he had to endure.

Another clue to Sadger's personality comes from a passage in Lou Andreas-Salome's (1861–1937) summary of the discussion following Sadger's presentation "On the Sadomasochistic Complex" given on November 6, 1912: "Freud had not much to say by way of concluding remarks, and he excused us all for being bored. He rightly supposed that if disgust with the topic did not itself create resistances, objective interest would have waned anyhow since the material, disgusting as it was, was also not meaningfully organized. But there is something about Sadger giving one the impression that it is not so much ability that he lacks as the desire to elevate the material through intellectual penetration from the unattractiveness of its crude content—as if in fact the demands of analysis disturbed his blissful contemplation. He presumably enjoys his analysands more than he helps them or learns anything from them" (Andreas-Salome 1987:41). Freud's actual remarks as reported in the minutes of the meeting included: "As to the paper itself, it is to be noted that the predominantly clinical material placed great demands upon the listeners and that the work lacks organization and structure" (Nunberg and Federn 1975:119).

Another analyst, Helene Deutsch (1884–1982), painted an even more disturbing portrait of Sadger. It is found in Roazen's biography of Deutsch. "Helene once remarked that at the first meeting of the society she attended, Isidor Sadger gave a paper on flowers in dreams; he had gone overboard in emphasizing the sexual themes that Freud had introduced and Sadger interpreted flowers as genital symbols. At the time Helene wondered to herself whether flowers could not also be just flowers. Among his Viennese adherents Freud put up with people he was dubious about. Sadger, for instance, had an almost pornographic interest in sex. (His own nails were dirty, and he would not even keep his analytic couch clean for a patient's head and feet.)" (Roazen 1985:150).

Another hint of Sadger's relationship to his patients is afforded by two passages in an exchange of letters between Freud and Ferenczi. Evidently a former patient of Ferenczi's from Pressburg had moved from Budapest to Vienna where he was being treated by Sadger. In a letter of April 12, 1910, Freud wrote Ferenczi, "Your young man from Pressburg is also dissatisfied here with Sadger; he likes you better as a person and he wants to go back to you. . . . I will take this opportunity to point out to you how wrong it is for you to charge ten crowns per session when Sadger demands twenty. You see, the ten didn't keep him with you and the twenty didn't keep him from going to Sadger." Ferenczi's answer, dated April 17, included: "The case of the young Pressburger is a wonderful case of *paranoia*. . . . The case is not suited to Sadger's somewhat coarse manner. The extraordinary role of projected homosexuality in paranoia is also confirmed here" (Brabant et al. 1992:161, 164).

Perhaps the most glaring anecdotal report of Sadger's alleged boorishness is found in a passage in Ernest Jones's autobiography. In describing the membership of the Wednesday Psychological Society before it had become the Vienna Psychoanalytic Society, Jones had this to say about Sadger: "Sadger was active at that time, and had not yet developed the curious reaction of mutism he displayed for some years before disappearing from the circle [Sadger resigned from the Society in 1933]. He was a morose, pathetic figure, very like a specially uncouth bear. One of his social gaffes was so terrific that it deserves recording. Seated at a Congress banquet next to a distinguished literary lady, he fumbled his way through the dinner, and finally ventured to address her.

His ever-memorable remark to this stranger was: 'Have you occupied yourself with masturbation?' one which in its German guise was even more ambiguous than in English" (1959:169).

What then do we know about Sadger? Despite his prolific writings, Sadger was never more than a minor figure in the development of psychoanalysis, though perhaps the rescue of this book from virtual oblivion may elevate his status to some degree. He is barely mentioned, if at all, in conventional histories of the psychoanalytic movement. One of the few relatively modern references to him refers to his having a "dutiful and unoriginal mind" (Lewes 1988:48). Yet he was one of the earliest students of Freud, attending his lectures at the University of Vienna and he was an active member, a very active member, of the Vienna Psychoanalytic Society. Sadger was a frequent participant in psychoanalytic congresses, including the very first one held in Salzburg in 1908 and the one in Oxford in 1929. In sheer terms of hours spent in the presence of Freud, including auditing his lectures, Sadger had few peers. Although members of Freud's inner circle did have the benefit of revealing correspondence with Freud, they did not live in Vienna—Abraham, Sachs, and Eitingon lived in Berlin, Ferenczi in Budapest, Jones in London (Sachs 1944:159).

Sadger did make some contributions to psychoanalytic theory. His application of psychoanalytic theory to homosexuality and particularly his suggestion that "narcissism" was related to the development of homo-sexuality influenced Freud. It is true that in a survey of the scholarship concerned with the psychoanalytic approach to homosexuality, the comment is made that early psychoanalysts such as Sadger "were not particu-larly distinguished and are virtually unknown today, except to specialists. In their rather large corpus of arti-cles on homosexuality, there is very little disagreement or original contribution. In fact, there is something rather touching in the careful piety of these workers in the field, gleaning in the train of their master" (Lewes 1988:48).

Although Sadger did not invent the term "narcis-sism" (May 1991), he is generally credited with intro-ducing it into psychoanalytic discourse (Pulver 1970; Reigstad 1980; Macmillan 1997:529). Sadger used the term in a paper (1908d) and on November 10, 1909, in the second segment of his three-part presentation "A Case of Multiform Perversion" when he remarked that "A large role is played by autoerotism in the form of narcissism" (Nunberg and Federn 1967:307). Freud's reaction to the presentation was typical: "The speaker did not succeed in mastering the material and in arriv-ing at a synthesis of the case." But he did give some praise: "Sadger's comment with regard to narcissism seems new and valuable" (312). In his comment on Sadger's presentation "On the Psychology of the Only

Child and the Favorite Child" on October 5, 1910, Freud agreed, "A prolonged remaining at the transitory stage of narcissism definitely predisposes to homosexuality" (Nunberg and Federn 1974:13). Freud later proceeded to expand upon the concept in several essays, including a footnote in his 1910 paper "Three Contributions to the Theory of Sex" and especially his 1914 paper "On Narcissism: An Introduction" (Gay 1988: 339; Henseller, 1991:195). Freud also gave credit to Sadger for the idea that all humans pass through an early bisexual stage in childhood, for example, in his 1909 "Analysis of a Phobia in a Five-Year-Old Boy" (1959a: 25In.1) and his 1920 "The Psychogenesis of a Case of Homosexuality in a Woman" (1959d:214). But in retrospect, possibly the most important contribution Sadger made was writing what may well be the first book-length evaluative review of Freud's life and work. It is a unique, perhaps unforgettable, portrait of Freud, unlike any other, a curious anecdotal mixture of extravagant hyperbolic praise and pointed, sometimes acerbic, criticisms. And it was written by—to modify the conventional anthropological idiom of "participant observer—an "observant participant" who was an eyewitness to the events he described. Why then has no one until now thought to consult it?

One reason for the failure of anyone to read Sadger's book is the fact that the few writers who even mention it believed the false rumor that it had never been published. Here is Roazen's account: "In his idolization of Freud, Jones did his best to suppress anything from being published about Freud which could be construed in an unflattering light. In the early 1930s Isidor Sadger, one of Freud's Vienna followers from before World War I, prepared a book on Freud; Jones was so incensed by some of the interpretations in it that he recommended in a letter to Federn that Sadger (who was Jewish) be put into a concentration camp, if need be, to make sure the book never appeared. (It was never published.)" (1976:351). Roazen cites as authority for this statement a letter from Jones to Federn, dated October 10, 1933. If Jones really did read the book, he must surely have been annoyed by Sadger's misspelling of his first name as well as that of Hanns Sachs, not to mention all the barbed criticisms of his idol Freud.

Vincent Brome in his biography of Jones gives a similar account: "Throughout the twenties and thirties Jones was busy attacking any book which criticized Freud or psycho-analysis, and one such book, by Isidor Sadger, so incensed him that he went beyond all normal limits in a letter to Federn. He suggested that if necessary Sadger—who was Jewish—should be put in a concentration camp to prevent the book appearing" (1983:186). Brome also cites a letter from Jones to Federn but gives the date as October 10, 1934. Lieberman in his biography of Rank notes the discrepancy in the date of the letter, 1933 versus 1934, adding that he had received a letter in 1984 from the son of Paul Federn indicating that he had no knowledge of such a letter to his father (1985:443n.15). Lieberman, however, notwithstanding the discrepancy repeats the false rumor: "In 1934, Jones was so upset with a manuscript written by the Viennese analyst Isidor Sadger that, in order to suppress it, he suggested Sadger be put in a concentration camp. (The suggestion was not followed, but neither was the manuscript published.)" (65).

None of these authors, apart from reiterating Jones's mean-spirited seemingly anti-Semitic remark, comment on the sad irony of it. For Sadger was in fact sent to the Theresienstadt concentration camp on September 10, 1942, where he died on the twentieth or twenty-first of December of that year (Mühlleitner 1992:283). Even Mühlleitner, who compiled a remarkably impressive set of capsule biographies of every single member of the Vienna Psychoanalytic Society, was taken in by the rumor. Claiming that Sadger's manuscript "Erinnerungen an Freud" had been written by the end of 1932, Mühlleitner says, "Das Manuskript wurde nicht publiziert und gilt als verschollen" (283, The manuscript was not published and must be considered as lost). Given this consensus, it is no wonder that no serious scholar, either a pro- or anti-Freudian would think about trying to find Sadger's book. There is something fishy about the rumor, however. Since the book was apparently published in 1930, it is not clear why Jones would be writing in either 1933 or 1934 urging that the book be suppressed.

The question remains, nevertheless, that if the book was actually published, why is it that no one, the above-mentioned false reports of it not being published notwithstanding, has managed to stumble upon a copy up to the present time? My own experience in connection with the book may shed some light on the answer to that question.

In the course of carrying out research on a psychoanalytic study of orthodox Jewish character (Dundes 2002), I had occasion to review the literature on anal erotic character. In re-reading the classic papers by Jones and Abraham, I realized I had never seen the early paper on the subject by Sadger in *Die Heilkunde,* cited favorably by both authors. When I looked up Sadger in my computer data base, I found not only the article in question but the title of a book: *Sigmund Freud: Persönliche Erinnerungen.* As I was not familiar with that work, I decided to send for it via interlibrary loan at the same time that I requested a copy of the anal erotic character paper. In due course, the latter arrived, but the effort to procure a copy of the former proved unsuccessful. I was informed that there was no known copy in the United States available for borrowing. Since I knew that the book had been published in Vienna, I asked if we could try to locate a copy in Europe and the obliging staff at interlibrary loan agreed to do so. A few weeks later, I learned that there was no known copy in any European library available for borrowing.

I was told, however, there was one, just one, copy listed that might be utilized and that copy was located in the library at Keio University in Japan. Again, interlibrary loan made a request on my behalf and this time with some partial success. Keio University library kindly sent a photocopy of the book's table of contents. The chapter titles looked intriguing: My First Encounter with Freud, Contributions to the Study of Freud's Character, Freud as Leader and Organizer, Freud's Wit, From the Last Years of Freud's Life, etc. I next asked interlibrary loan to request a photocopy of the entire book, indicating that I was more than willing to pay the cost of such. In February of 2001 my effort to obtain a photocopy hit a snag. The Keio University Mita Media Center informed our interlibrary loan office that it was unable to comply with my request. "This is because photocopying of this book is limited by the copyright law." I did not then, nor do I now understand this reason for the refusal to photocopy the book. First of all, the book was published in Vienna, not in Japan, and secondly, the period of copyright had long since expired. Still, I was, for the moment, stymied.

As it happened, one of my anthropology doctoral students, Hideaki Matsuoka, had just finished his degree and was returning to his native Japan. I asked him to do me a big favor and get me a photocopy of the book. He first tried to do so via interlibrary loan from his university, Tokyo Woman's Christian University, but to no avail. As only students and faculty at Keio University were permitted to use books in its library, he had to get a special letter of introduction from his university in order to have access to the book. Then he went to Keio University where he personally made a photocopy. A few weeks later, I found a photocopy of Sadger's book in my mailbox. I then asked one of my former students, Johanna Micaela Jacobsen, a doctoral student in folklore and folklife at the University of Pennsylvania, to undertake a preliminary translation of the book and she was kind enough to do so.

I mention all this to explain why even if someone did know that Sadger's book was published, it would not be all that easy to find a copy to read. As to the reason why the book is in so few libraries, one can only speculate. In view of Jones's alleged hostility to the book and his hope that the book would be suppressed, one is tempted to speculate that pro-Freudians might have taken Jones's request seriously and purchased as many copies of the original book as possible in order to destroy them. The book does not even seem to be included in the official list of books contained in Freud's personal library. But this kind of conspiracy theory seems unlikely.

There is one final question that must be raised and that is: Why should a book on Freud dating from 1930 be translated now in the twenty-first century, almost seventy-five years after it was first published? There are few, if any, new facts about Freud's life that are not already well-known and documented by countless other books. Psychoanalytic theory has changed considerably since 1930, as both advocates and critics can attest. It would take an extensive set of editorial footnotes to update all the topics covered by Sadger in the light of all the biographies of Freud published since 1930 and all the advances and criticisms of psychoanalytic theory and practice during the same period. And what about Sadger's own problematic relationship to Freud? Given Freud's attitude towards Sadger, not to mention the attitudes of other members of the Vienna Psychoanalytic Society regarding Sadger, what credence should legitimately be placed in Sadger's recollections of Freud?

It seems to me that Sadger's unique position as a very early disciple of Freud but who was not one of Freud's intimate friends makes his account of Freud invaluable. Most of those writing about Freud in modern times never knew Freud personally and never even met him. Sadger, in contrast, knew Freud over a period of thirty-five years and spent many hours in his immediate presence. Whatever his bias might have been and however much he may have chafed under the ceaseless criticism offered by Freud and others, Sadger had a rare opportunity to observe Freud in action at close quarters, often in Freud's own home. For this reason alone, his take on Freud is worth making available to partisans and Freud-bashers alike. Freud was not a perfect human being, as he would probably have been the first to acknowledge. Sadger in his own fashion tries to present in a clear and forthright manner what he considers to be both the positive and negative aspects of Freud's character. In that sense, his recollections of Freud may provide a useful bridge between the hagiographic accounts by Ernest Jones and others and the poisonous vilifications penned by Freud-haters. Surely there is some value, even after so many years, in Sadger's *Recollecting Freud*. (I have taken some editorial liberties with the original title but have otherwise tried to remain faithful to the original text. Bracketed items are my editorial additions while parenthetical remarks are Sadger's few footnotes inserted into the text. Extended quotations from Freud's writings are indented.) As a document describing an important period in human history, it certainly deserves to be available to anyone with a serious interest in Freud and/or the history of psychoanalysis (*pace* Ernest Jones).

References

Abraham, Hilda C. 1974. *Karl Abraham: biographie inachevée*. Paris: Presses Universitaires de France.

Abraham, Karl. 1953. Contributions to the Theory of the Anal Character. In *Selected Papers on Psychoanalysis*. 370–392. New York: Basic Books.

Andreas-Salome, Lou. 1987. *The Freud Journal*. London: Quartet Books.

Anthi, Per Roar. 1990. Freud's Dream in Norekdal Style. *The Scandinavian Psychoanalytic Review* 13:138–160.

Balmary, Marie. 1982. *Psychoanalyzing Psychoanalysis. Freud and the Hidden Fault of the Father*. Baltimore: The Johns Hopkins University Press.

Berthelslen, Detlef. 1987. *Alltag bei Familie Freud: die Erinnerungen der Paula Fichtl*. Hamburg: Hoffmann und Campe.

Binswanger, Ludwig. 1957. *Sigmund Freud: Reminiscences of a Friendship*. New York: Grune & Stratton.

Blanton, Smiley. 1971. *Diary of My Analysis with Sigmund Freud*. New York: Hawthorn Books.

Brabant, Eva, Ernst Falzeder, and Patrizia Giampieri-Deutsch, eds. 1992. *The Correspondence of Sigmund Freud and Sándor Ferenczi, Volume I, 1908–1914*. Cambridge: Harvard University Press.

Brill, Abraham Arden. 1940. Reflections, Reminiscences of Sigmund Freud. *Medical Leaves* 3:18–29.

Brome, Vincent. 1983. *Ernest Jones: Freud's Alter Ego*. New York: W. W. Norton.

Clark, Ronald W. 1980. *Freud, the Man and the Cause: A Biography*. New York: Random House.

Crews, Frederick C., ed. 1998. *Unauthorized Freud: Doubters Confront a Legend*. New York: Viking.

D[oolittle], H[ilda]. 1984. *Tribute to Freud, by H.D.* New York: New Directions Books.

Dolnick, Edward. 1998. *Madness on the Couch: Blaming the Victim in the Heyday of Psychoanalysis*. New York: Simon and Schuster.

Dorsey, John M. 1976. *An American Psychiatrist in Vienna, 1935–1937, and His Sigmund Freud*. Detroit: Center for Health Education.

Dufresne, Todd. 1996. An Interview with Joseph Wortis. *Psychoanalytic Review* 83:589–610.

Dundes, Alan. 2002. *The Shabbat Elevator and Other Sabbath Subterfuges: An Unorthodox Essay on Circumventing Custom and Jewish Character*. Lanham, Md.: Rowman & Littlefield.

Ferris, Paul. 1997. *Dr. Freud: A Life*. Washington, D.C.: Counterpoint.

Fine, Reuben. 1979. *A History of Psychoanalysis*. New York: Columbia University Press.

Freud, Ernst L., ed. 1975. *The Letters of Sigmund Freud*. New York: Basic Books.

Freud, Martin. 1957. *Glory Reflected: Sigmund Freud—Man and Father*. London: Angus and Robertson.

Freud, Sigmund. 1905. Three Essays on the Theory of Sexuality. Vol. 7 of *The Standard Edition*. 123–245. London: Hogarth Press.

———. 1908. Hysterical Phantasies and Their Relations to Bisexuality. Vol. 9 of *The Standard Edition*. 155–166. London: Hogarth Press.

———. 1910. Leonardo Da Vinci and A Memory of His Childhood. Vol. 11 of *The Standard Edition*. 57–137. London: Hogarth Press.

———. 1920. A Case of Homosexuality in a Woman. Vol. 18 of *The Standard Edition*. 147–172. London: Hogarth Press.

———. 1938. *The Basic Writings of Sigmund Freud*. New York: The Modern Library.

———. 1959a. Analysis of a Phobia in a Five-Year-Old Boy (1909). Vol. 3 of *Collected Papers*. New York: Basic Books.

———. 1959b. On Narcissism: An Introduction (1914). Vol. 4 of *Collected Papers*. 30–59. New York: Basic Books.

———. 1959c. Psycho-Analytic Notes upon an Autobiographical Account of a Case of Paranoia (Dementia Paranoides) (1911). Vol. 3 of *Collected Papers*. 387–470. New York: Basic Books.

———. 1959d. The Psychogenesis of a Case of Homosexuality in a Woman (1920). Vol. 2 of *Collected Papers*. New York: Basic Books.

Friedländer, A. 1911. Hysteria and Modern Psychoanalysis. *Journal of Abnormal Psychology* 5:297–319.

Gay, Peter. 1988. *Freud: A Life for Our Time*. New York: W. W. Norton.

Goetz, Bruno. 1969. *Erinnerungen an Sigmund Freud*. Berlin: Friedenauer Presse.

Graf, Max. 1942. Reminiscences of Professor Sigmund Freud. *Psychoanalytic Quarterly* 11:465–476.

Grinker, Roy R. 1940. Reminiscences of a Personal Contact with Freud. *American Journal of Orthopsychiatry* 10:850–854.

Gross, Edith B. 1979. Psychoanalysis as an Emerging Specialty: A Sociological Study of the Vienna Psychoanalytic Society. *Journal of the Philadelphia Association for Psychoanalysis* 6:163–174.

Grosskurth, Phyllis. 1991. *The Secret Ring: Freud's Inner Circle and the Politics of Psychoanalysis.* Reading, Mass.: Addison-Wesley Publishing Company.

Handlbauer, Bernhard. 1998. *The Freud-Adler Controversy.* Oxford: One World.

Henseller, Heinz. 1991. Narcissism as a Form of Relationship. In *Freud's "On Narcissism: An Introduction.* Edited by Joseph Sandler, Ethel Spector Person, and Peter Fonagy. 195–215. New Haven: Yale University Press.

Jones, Ernest. 1953, 1955, 1957. *The Life and Work of Sigmund Freud.* 3 vols. New York: Basic Books.

———. 1959. *Free Associations: Memoirs of a Psychoanalyst.* New York: Basic Books.

———. 1961. Anal-Erotic Character Traits. In *Papers on Psycho-Analysis.* 413–437. Boston: Beacon Press.

Kardiner, A. 1977. *My Analysis with Freud: Reminiscences.* New York: W. W. Norton.

Kiell, Norman. 1988. *Freud without Hindsight: Reviews of His Work (1893–1939).* Madison, Conn.: International Universities Press.

Lewes, Kenneth. 1988. *The Psychoanalytic Theory of Male Homosexuality.* New York: Simon and Schuster.

Lieberman, E. James. 1985. *Acts of Will: The Life and Work of Otto Rank*. New York: The Free Press.

Macmillan, Malcolm. 1997. *Freud Evaluated: The Completed Arc*. Cambridge: MIT Press.

Masson, Jeffrey Moussaieff, ed. 1985. *The Complete Letters of Sigmund Freud to Wilhelm Fliess, 1887–1904*. Cambridge: Harvard University Press.

May, Ulrike. 1991. Zu den Anfängen des Narzissimus. Ellis—Näcke—Sadger—Freud. *Luzifer-Amor: Zeitschrift zur Geschichte der Psychoanalyse* 4:50–88.

———. 1999. Ein Traum (1897) und ein Brief (1902): Zur frühen Beziehung zwischen Freud und Isidor Sadger. *Luzifer-Amor: Zeitschrift zur Geschichte der Psychoanalyse* 12:25–48.

———. 2003. The Early Relationship Between Sigmund Freud and Isidor Sadger: A Dream (1897) and a Letter (1902). *Psychoanalysis & History* 5: 119–145.

McGuire, William, ed. 1974. *The Freud–Jung Letters*. Princeton: Princeton University Press.

Meng, Heinrich, and Ernst L. Freud, eds. 1963. *Psychoanalysis and Faith: The Letters of Sigmund Freud and Oskar Pfister*. New York: Basic Books.

Mitchell, Stephen A., and Margaret J. Black. 1995. *Freud and Beyond: A History of Modern Psychoanalytic Thought*. New York: Basic Books.

Mühlleitner, Elke. 1992. *Biographisches Lexikon der Psychoanalyse: Die Mitglieder der Psychologischen*

Mittwoch-Gesellschaft und der Wiener Psychoanalytischen Vereinigung 1902–1938. Tübingen: Edition diskord.

———. 2000. Frauen in der Psychoanalytischen Bewegung. Der Fall der Wiener Psychoanalytischen Vereinigung 1902–1938. *Psyche* (Stuttgart) 54:642–668.

Mühlleitner, Elke, and Johannes Reichmayr. 1998. Die Freudianer in Wien. Die Psychologische Mittwoch-Gesellschaft und die Wiener Psychoanalytische Vereinigung 1902–1938. *Psyche* (Stuttgart) 51:1051–1103.

Niederland, William G. 1974. *The Schreber Case: Psychoanalytic Profile of a Paranoid Personality*. New York: Quadrangle.

Nunberg, Herman, and Ernst Federn. 1962. *Minutes of the Vienna Psychoanalytic Society, Volume I: 1906–1908*. New York: International Universities Press.

———. 1967. *Minutes of the Vienna Psychoanalytic Society, Volume II: 1908–1910*. New York: International Universities Press.

———. 1974. *Minutes of the Vienna Psychoanalytic Society, Volume III: 1910–1911*. New York: International Universities Press.

———. 1975. *Minutes of the Vienna Psychoanalytic Society, Volume IV: 1912–1918*. New York: International Universities Press.

Paskauskas, R. Andrew, ed. 1993. *The Complete Correspondence of Sigmund Freud and Ernest Jones, 1908–1939*. Cambridge: Harvard University Press.

Pouh, Lieselotte. 2000. *Young Vienna and Psychoanalysis*. New York: Peter Lang.

Pulver, Sydney E. 1970. Narcissism: The Term and the Concept. *Journal of the American Psychoanalytic Association* 18:319–342.

Reichmayr, Johannes. 1995. New Biographical Research on the Members of the Psychoanalytic Movement in Vienna 1902–1938. *International Forum of Psychoanalysis* 4:179–183.

Reigstad, Ståle. 1980. Utviklingen av narsissismebegrepet i psychoanalytic teori. *Tidsskrift for Norsk Psykologforening* 17:286–291.

Reik, Theodor. 1940. *From Thirty Years with Freud*. New York: Farrar & Rinehart.

Roazen, Paul. 1976. *Freud and His Followers*. New York: Knopf.

———. 1985. *Helene Deutsch: A Psychoanalyst's Life*. Garden City, N.Y.: Anchor Press.

———. 1995. *How Freud Worked*. Northvale, N.J.: Jason Aronson.

———. 2001. *The Historiography of Psychoanalysis*. New Brunswick, N.J.: Transaction Publishers.

Robinson, Paul. 1993. *Freud and His Critics*. Berkeley: University of California Press.

———. 2000. Freud and Homosexuality. In *Whose Freud? The Place of Psychoanalysis in Contemporary Culture*. Edited by Peter Brooks and Alex Woloch. 144–149. New Haven: Yale University Press.

Rose, Louis. 1998. *The Freudian Calling: Early Viennese Psychoanalysis and the Pursuit of Cultural Science.* Detroit: Wayne State University Press.

Ruitenbeek, Hendrik M., ed. 1973. *Freud as We Knew Him.* Detroit: Wayne State University Press.

Sachs, Hanns. 1944. *Freud: Master and Friend.* Cambridge: Harvard University Press.

Sadger, Isidor. 1896a. Die Ärzte und die Kaltwasserkuren. *Blätter für klinische Hydrotherapie* 6: 127–134.

———. 1896b. Die Lehrnotwendigkeit der Hydrotherapie. *Blätter für klinische Hydrotherapie* 6: 217–222.

———. 1897. Das Wunder vom denkenden Eiweiss. *Deutsche Revue* 22:93–110.

———. 1907. Die Bedeutung der psychoanalytischen Methode nach Freud. *Centralblatt für Nervenheilkunde und Psychiatrie* 30:41–52.

———. 1908a. Fragment der Psychoanalyse eines Homosexuellen. *Jahrbuch für sexuelle Zwischenstufen unter besonderer Berücksichtigung der Homosexualität* 9:339–424.

———. 1908b. Ist die konträre Sexualempfindung heilbar? *Zeitschrift für Sexualwissenschaft* 712–720.

———. 1908c. *Konrad Ferdinand Meyer. Ein pathographisch-psychologische Studie.* Wiesbaden: Bergmann.

———. 1908d. Psychiatrisch-Neurologisches in Psychoanalytischer Beleuchtung. *Zentralblatt für die*

Gesamtgebiet der *Medizin und ihrer Hilfswissenschaften* 4 (7):45–47, 53–57.

——. 1909a. *Aus dem Liebesleben Nikolaus Lenau.* Leipzig: Deuticke.

——. 1909b. Zur Ätiologie der konträren Sexualempfindung. *Medizinische Klinik* 5:53–56.

——. 1910a. Analerotik und Analcharakter. *Die Heilkunde* 43–46.

——. 1910b. Heinrich von Kleist. Eine pathologischpsychologische Studie. Wiesbaden: J. F. Bergmann.

——. 1910c. Über Urethralerotik. *Jahrbuch der Psychoanalyse* 2:409–450.

——. 1911. Die Traumdeutung. *Anthropophyteia Jahrbücher* 8:489–490.

——. 1912. Von der Pathographie zur Psychographie. *Imago* 1:158–175.

——. 1913a. Über Gesässerotik. *Internationale Zeitschrift für ärztliche Psychoanalyse* 1:351–358.

——. 1913b. Über den sado-masochistischen Komplex. *Jahrbuch der Psychoanalyse* 5:157–232.

——. 1913c. Welcher Wert kommt den Erzählungen und Autobiographien der Homosexuellen zu? *Archiv für Kriminal-Anthropologie und Kriminalistik* 53:179–187.

——. 1920a. *Friedrich Hebbel, ein psychoanalytischer Versuch.* Vienna: Deuticke.

——. 1920b. *Sleep Walking and Moon Walking: A Medico-Literary Study.* New York: Nervous and Mental Disease Publishing Company.

———. 1921. *Die Lehre von den Geschlechtsverwirrungen* (Psychopathia sexualis) *auf psychoanalytischer Grundlage.* Leipzig and Vienna: Deuticke.

———. 1926. A Contribution to the Understanding of Sado-Masochism. *The International Journal of Psycho-Analysis* 7:484–491.

———. 1927. Comment. *The International Journal of Psycho-Analysis* 8:274.

———. 1929. Genital and Extragenital Libido. *The International Journal of Psycho-Analysis* 10:348–356.

———. 1930. *Sigmund Freud: Persönliche Erinnerungen.* Vienna: Ernst Wengraf Verlag.

Schorske, Carl E. 1980. *Fin-de-siècle Vienna: Politics and Culture.* New York: Knopf.

Schreber, Daniel Paul. 1903. *Denkwürdigkeiten eines Nervenkranken.* Leipzig: O. Mutze.

Schur, Max. 1972. *Freud: Living and Dying.* New York: International Universities Press.

Schwartz, Joseph. 1999. *Cassandra's Daughter: A History of Psychoanalysis.* New York: Viking.

Sharaf, Myron. 1983. *Fury on Earth: A Biography of Wilhelm Reich.* New York: St. Martin's Press.

Stekel, Wilhelm. 1950. *The Autobiography of Wilhelm Stekel: The Life Story of a Pioneer Psychoanalyst.* New York: Liveright.

Sterba, Richard F. 1982. *Reminiscences of a Viennese Psychoanalyst.* Detroit: Wayne State University Press.

Stern, Adolph. 1922. Some Personal Psychoanalytical

Experiences with Prof. Freud. *New York State Journal of Medicine* 22:21–25.

Thornton, E. M. 1984. *The Freudian Fallacy.* Garden City, N.Y.: Doubleday.

Torrey, E. Fuller. 1992. *Freudian Fraud: The Malignant Effect of Freud's Theory on American Thought and Culture.* New York: HarperCollins.

Von Urban, Rudolf. 1958. *Myself Not Least: A Confessional Autobiography of a Psychoanalyst and Some Explanatory History Cases.* London: Jarrolds.

Webster, Richard. 1995. *Why Freud Was Wrong.* New York: Basic Books.

Weiss, Edoardo. 1970. *Sigmund Freud as a Consultant: Recollections of a Pioneer in Psychoanalysis.* New York: Intercontinental Medical Book Corporation.

Wittels, Fritz. 1924. *Sigmund Freud: His Personality, His Teaching, and His School.* New York: Dodd, Mead & Company.

———. 1931. *Freud and His Time.* New York: Grosset & Dunlap.

———. 1995. *Freud and the Child Woman: The Memoirs of Fritz Wittels.* Edited by Edward Timms. New Haven: Yale University Press.

Wortis, Joseph. 1940. Fragments of a Freudian Analysis. *American Journal of Orthopsychiatry* 10:843–849.

———. 1954. *Fragments of an Analysis with Freud.* New York: Simon and Schuster.

Recollecting Freud

Fortunate is the man who feels foreign greatness
And who makes it his own through love.

Grillparzer

Preface

I reserve the right in these purely personal recollections to show the whole of Freud in all of his extraordinary genius as well as in his mistakes. I am well aware of the danger that critics may simply pounce upon the latter. They would see only the vulnerable spot on the totality of Achilles, his heel! But no one is immune from malicious criticism. And perhaps it is this obsessive attempt to belittle a scholar using any means available that is precisely the proof of that scholar's importance. Were he not so great, who would take the trouble to seek to make him less so? There is one more thing that I would like to add: The following chapters contain nothing other than what I personally experienced, and the impressions that Freud's character, his actions and his writing made on me. In no place have I sought to present biographical details that I did not myself witness.

My First Encounter
with Freud

It was in September of 1895 that my recently deceased colleague Dr. Max Kahane [1866–1923] approached me with the question of whether I might not want to attend the lectures on psychoneuroses scheduled to be given by Docent Sigmund Freud. I had little enthusiasm for the prospect of doing so. Up until that time, I had read only a very interesting but hardly epoch-making study on aphasia by Freud and I had heard further that as an assistant to [Theodor] Meynert [1833–1892], he had, with the help of a government stipend, gone to France and had translated the lectures of [Jean Martin] Charcot [1825–1893] and [Hippolyte] Bernheim [1840–1919] into German.

More than that about him, I did not know nor had I yet at that time made his personal acquaintance. Finally, my respect for clinical assistants in psychiatry was never very great and totally psychiatric periodicals or even books seemed to me something that God could only have put into the world in His greatest wrath. If these two types of publications were not named among the plagues of Egypt, it is only because God Himself did not think of such plagues during the times of the blessed Pharaoh.

So it was that I didn't exactly respond to Kahane's suggestion with shouts of joy. It required repeated pressure and prodding on Kahane's part until I finally decided to register for Freud's lectures. Dr. Max Kahane, Dr. Isidor Fischer, gynecologist and current Docent for the history of medicine, and finally yours truly were the first three students to be introduced to Freud's theory of neuroses. To be more precise, in the winter semester of 1895–1896, Freud covered neurasthenia and anxiety neuroses; in the summer semester of 1896, hysteria and compulsive neuroses. Of these three auditors, Max Kahane soon devoted himself almost entirely to physical therapy, Dr. Fischer up until the present day works only as a gynecologist and never practiced psychoanalysis, so that I can justifiably claim to be the oldest at the very least among the practicing students of Freud.

I would not mention all these circumstances in such great detail had Freud not fully "repressed" the recollection of that first set of lectures in his "History of the Psychoanalytic Movement" together with many other details which were, so to speak, erased from his memory. This genius had, moreover, among his great intellectual gifts also the invaluable capacity of being able to completely forget entirely unpleasant matters. These include the fact that he started from such small beginnings, that the three who first attended his lectures had to be drummed up with great difficulty and furthermore that this was done by one of them [Kahane] with whom he would later have a falling out. This was to his way of thinking not a happy memory.

For a great man who has worked his way up from humble origins, there are two possibilities: Either he places his tattered boots with which he marched into town under a glass dome and tells everyone, "In these tattered boots I came into town and now I am a great man!" or he never had to wear torn boots in the first place. Freud never had such boots; he was a great man from the very beginning.

But now back to the first set of lectures. Freud began his lecture with a critical review of the state of knowledge about neurasthenia and hysteria, not failing to note the lack of success of the current healing treatments. What he presented every thinking neurologist must have already said to himself and at most his precise and sparkling formulations were highly engaging. Still, criticizing one's predecessors is always the easiest part of any science. After this striking critical introduction, I was eager to know what new ideas would be set forth. And then there actually came something truly amazing. I heard for the first time that there were specific and decisive sexual causes of psychoneuroses, more particularly that actual harmful injury was related to neurasthenia and anxiety neuroses, and on the other hand, infantile psychological factors were determinants of hysteria and compulsive neuroses. Freud then elaborated these ideas using examples from individual cases in his practice.

It was now necessary to test these amazing new notions with the very same critical acuity that Freud himself had employed with respect to earlier scientific views. This was relatively easy to accomplish through actual neuroses by means of which one could directly test therapeutic efficacy. Here the results were often truly astonishing and since one could, with a knowledge of etiology, quickly and without difficulty eliminate the harmful cause, this portion of Freudian doctrine was even accepted by mainstream neurology without further difficulty. Even today, in investigating cases of severe anxiety, one dares to ask whether perhaps inappropriate means were utilized to prevent conception and a privy councilor is even said to have boldly asked a sweet eighteen-year-old girl whether or not she masturbated.

It was more difficult to verify the approaches to hysteria and compulsive neuroses, especially because the technique of the procedure, even for the discoverer, was, so to speak, still in swaddling clothes. *The Interpretation of Dreams* did not yet exist at that time. Nor did *Three Essays on the Theory of Sexuality* and there was no knowledge of the Oedipus and Castration complexes, nor of Narcissism, guilt feelings, and the super-ego. At best, one spoke of hysterical patients suffering from diminished affect, conversion, abreaction, and memory. If one had, as I did, quite the bad luck to get among the first cases the most desperate ones, for example, the most severe compulsive neuroses that had lasted for years—and at that time only other equally desperate cases were willing to undergo psychoanalytic treatment—it becomes understandable that one was not always prepared to deal with them. Nevertheless, I was satisfied with my results, especially if I compared the successes of psychoanalysis with the outcomes of other conventional methods such as bromine and opium, electricity and water cures, hypnosis, and so-called psychotherapy, methods that in spite of many applications in complicated cases failed completely.

I need to make several additional observations about the style and character of those first lectures. At that time, since there was still too much groping, tentativeness, and uncertainty in the study of psycho-neuroses, Freud's expressions were not a breath of fresh air, were not marked by the classic simplicity that would characterize his later papers. At any rate, many features were enjoyable and one was not used to hearing such from clinics. What was missing, first of all, was all that psychiatric gibberish, all that scrambling after new technical terminology that only the initiated could understand and by which experts can recognize one another, just as the Roman Augurs did to the extent that they would be provoked to the point of laughter. If it can be said about anything, one could legitimately describe modern psychiatry as a misuse of its own private terminology, invented for this very purpose.

This difference between Freud and most other scientists I will illustrate with one single example, one that doesn't even involve a psychiatrist. When [Josef] Breuer [1842–1925] and Freud first considered the question of the psychological mechanism of hysteria, Breuer created the theory of "hypnoid states" while Freud interpreted the mental breakdown of the hysteric as the result of a "defense," later called "repression." In this departure from any foreign language nomenclature, there lies more than just simple purism. "Oh, what a poor language German is! What a crude language!" says Riccaut de la Marlinière. If a scientist wants to conceal the lack of clarity in his thought, wants to keep anyone from noticing how little he has achieved in reaching the solution to a problem's questions, he will first of all, with the help of a Latin or Greek dictionary, preferably invent a new technical expression, if possible, one that is totally unprecedented. In contrast, one who still uses pure German words will be compelled by this means alone to achieve maximum clarity and comprehension. One notices on the spot in the German turn of phrase if something hovers not fully formed in the mind of the discoverer. A thing can be said in straightforward German or in fraudulent gibberish. Freud was a master from the start, precisely in his choice of appropriate, lucid, instantly grasped technical terms.

In addition to this clarity and overall intelligibility, Freud's lectures had still other good qualities that one seldom finds so felicitously combined. Above all, he had an unrelentingly sharp logic that was not intimidated by any authority and furthermore an ever-ready wit, especially employed against adversaries who were always endeavoring to quash his genius by a failure to understand the "closely packed body of material." If to this remarkable pedagogical talent that could in and of itself introduce the most difficult trains of thought with ease, we add finally, as well, his specific dialectic that anticipated and refuted every possible objection and opposition, then one will understand the great charisma that Freud already exhibited in his first lectures in the year 1895, a charisma that increased ever more with the passing years. None of my other university professors could, by way of example, have easily reiterated all of the basic principles to me always with refreshing delight, to transmit the system of knowledge concerning psychoneuroses over a period of twenty-two years, each time from a different angle, always with new unfolding perceptions. In what follows, I will have occasion to further clarify these qualities in more detail.

Freud as Speaker and Writer, Stylist and Critic

In the previous chapter, I described the impression that the first lectures of Freud made on me at a point in time when he was engaged in his earliest exploratory writings and everything was still in a stage of development. So now I will sketch the professor during the time of the height of his intellectual powers when his wisdom generated new annual tree-rings from one moment to the next. To listen to Freud was in and of itself sheer pleasure. He spoke simply and plainly in an everyday fashion, as if in a private two-party face-to-face conversation. Never did I hear from him a trite phrase—unless it was an expression of condolence. He lacked all traces of pathos and every high-flying rhetorical flourish that experienced speakers were able to easily fabricate in order to make a good exit line. Only now and then did a couple flashes of humor suddenly illuminate a problem. For Freud, Goethe's words never held true: "It is only the lecture that accounts for the speaker's luck." Quite the contrary. His deepest insights were stated almost conversationally, not as a professor *ex cathedra,* nor as a flashy orator. Rather they came as if from a contemplative thinker whose thoughts were slowly released from his soul. At all times factual and objective, he made a point of avoiding any deception. When he was merely trying to persuade, he chose almost exclusively German expressions, even for the most difficult trains of thought, demonstrating a masterful command of language. He was not interested so much in the momentary effect but rather in presenting the truth and in being understood. There was also no feigning of pretended profundity, no colorful linguistic terminology, comprehensible to only the most initiated few. Instead, insights were dropped, as it were, in conversation. I have never known anyone else who knew how to say such deep things in the most light, conversational manner.

I always found admirable his knack of playfully introducing listeners to even the most theoretical material. A critic once spoke quite aptly of Freud's "irresistible pedagogy." Of what did this knack consist? I believe it was based on two different teaching techniques. First of all, the professor knew how to make his listeners think that they already understood all the things that he had just creatively presented to them for the first time so that it somehow felt as though he had not actually taught them anything new at all. This was clearly a trait of someone with a fine-tuned knowledge of human nature. Generally speaking, people do not tend to think that someone else is smarter than they hold themselves to be. On the contrary, as soon as such a thought enters their consciousness, they become extremely angry. It is quite annoying to have to become acquainted with new ideas; one could almost say it was an unreasonable impertinence to be asked to do so. He who puts new things, presumably truths, into my brain violates not merely the eternal brazen law of idleness, and not only scares me out of my well deserved rest, but even worse, he lays claim to being smarter and a deeper thinker than my own magnificent self. This leads naturally to everyone's narcissism erupting, especially if contrasted with an as yet unrecognized greatness.

Freud approached these things quite differently. One example may stand for many. At the Psychoanalytic Congress in Berlin [September 1922, the last of these congresses attended by Freud], he presented for the first time, publicly, the concept of "unconscious guilt-feelings." But how carefully, with what calculation of human frailty, did he do so. As always, it began with his familiar playing to the narcissism of his listeners. "You know," he would begin, "we distinguish between a Conscious and an Unconscious. That you all know, of course!" The listener would feel quite pleased with himself. "And then we distinguish in the Unconscious an uppermost layer, the Preconscious, which without further treatment can become conscious, and a repressed Unconscious that we have to first, with some effort, bring to light through our psychoanalytic method. But you all know that as well!" There is absolute assent by the entire audience; their sense of well-being soars. What a truly enjoyable speaker! "And then we also have an unconscious guilt feeling which often controls our actions to a very wide extent. But you all know that too!" Two minutes earlier, certainly no one in the entire circle had known any of this, yet since the Professor had so benevolently assumed that all those present had such knowledge, one had to think that one must already have known this in some corner of his mind. This was also highly supportive, unconsciously, to one's own sense of superiority. And inasmuch as one had already known these things all along, there was no real reason to disagree. On the contrary, one was thrilled with oneself and believed this to be a result of the new teachings. Talking to oneself after these so effective intellectual introductions removed just the instinctive opposition, the hatred of the new, of proselytism, not the contradiction of reason.

A second characteristic of Freud's pedagogy consisted in the fact that he always sought to anticipate any possible objection, by saying it himself and immediately rebutting it before the listener could even have time to think about it. (A striking example of this can be found in the first chapter of the *Introductory Lectures on Psychoanalysis,* spoken more or less in the same way as it is now presented in written form.) Moreover, the Professor demonstrated that he was so much more intelligent than those present, raising objections that no one had thought of, and, in a way, showing them how smart and wise they could have been. On the other hand, however, he took care not to play the part of a fault-finding genius bringing their inferiority to consciousness. Rather, he spoke always, as it were, as a representative of the audience in which everyone was just as smart as the lecturer himself. And again everyone present in the group felt edified by their own wisdom.

The above was an attempt to present Freud's innate ability to teach, the intuitive pedagogy he exhibited, which he took care to utilize in his lectures. Though at hand were, to be sure, such means fit to effectively neutralize objections from the outset, stemming from vulnerable narcissism and a state of mental laziness. However, these means were not what made his essays delightful reading, which they were in truth for everyone. There is yet one more decisive additional factor that I will now discuss in more detail.

All his life, Freud was reflective and speculative—I almost want to say he was compulsive in nature—and he had, as such, always a lot to say. What was more important is that he was not just merely reflective, he was, over and above that, a genius, that is, he usually had the right idea, or if he did not hit the bull's-eye, he would at least have hit the nearest concentric circle and then hit the center on the second shot. If, however, he once in a while appeared to miss the mark, as originally was the case with compulsive neurosis, it did not stop him from ten years later going all the way back to begin anew to finally find the solution on the basis of much more experience. On a walk years ago, he once told me how he had found one key after another to the understanding of hysteria. And in conversation, he once remarked, "If one approaches a thing without preconceptions, then one will find something." He also liked to quote the words of Charcot: "One has to look at things for a long time and over and over again until they begin to tell you something." But for them to tell you the correct thing, to be sure, one must be not only reflective, but also a genius, especially in so difficult a field as psychiatry.

However, from Freud, we have also learned never to be satisfied with just one solution. In psychiatric matters, one must always look for layers and for different forces struggling with one another. The master taught that "Clarity is in science always a falsification! Truth is always complicated and not particularly obvious!" Obvious and clear, things became persuasive at first mostly when tamed by Freud's presentation. And then at its best in a live lecture, not when he was at his desk condensing material for publication. After he had spoken flawlessly for nearly two hours at his Saturday lecture, there was literally no more doubt and no lack of understanding.

Yet even more significant, however, are my memories of the circle of intimates at the Wednesday evening meetings, the first of which were then still held in the home of the Professor himself. To hear the Professor lecture there on some new discovery, to some extent in *statu nascendi,* belongs to the most memorable experiences of my life. I cannot describe the impression as anything other than overwhelming. Ever since my student days, I have always been attracted to genius, though that certainly is very rarely found among those holding academic positions. I have listened to several very different geniuses, receiving from them a variety of impressions, for example, from the lectures of Theodor Meynert, the teacher of Freud. To listen to his lecture for three-quarters of an hour was one of the most exhausting experiences one could imagine. He spoke in a condensed manner, to an extreme degree, and, in addition, not infrequently in twisted turns of phrase. One could sense the breath of genius, but at the end of such a lecture one was worn out. Truthfully, one had to struggle for the pleasure by the sweat of one's brow.

It was also not always easy to listen to Freud. On those occasions when Freud had stored up his knowledge for a long time, he would give such a profusion of detail that a normal brain could no longer accommodate it. I remember, for example, a lecture on compulsive neurosis when Freud spoke for no less than three hours. Now, the listener's capacity for absorbing is ultimately limited. One could follow for the first two hours in spite of the fact that one was overwhelmed in due course with new viewpoints and outlooks, and one had great difficulty even in hastily taking in the materials presented. In the third hour my brain failed. It was not Freud who failed, because I believe that this genius could have continued to speak all night in such a fashion, still presenting ever new materials. Only where to put this tremendous rich harvest? Here one could only listen with one's ears and let the overflow wash over on oneself. Later Freud presented the same subject, though in essentially abridged form, at the first psychoanalytic congress in Salzburg [April 26, 1908]. It was again something different with many new things, though not with the superabundance of insights as that time in Vienna. Still, it nevertheless made an overwhelming impression on such inflexible and critical individuals as Eugen Bleuler [1857–1939] and C. G. Jung [1875–1961]. And finally the topic was put before us for a third time, namely in print. This now compressed the topic into a completely condensed form, packed with insight, but without the magic of his inspiring spoken words.

It was also highly enthralling to listen to Freud in discussion. There was no better, more insightful, and no more convincing critic than he, that is, if he chose to be critical. Time and time again, the following observation could be made. For hours, the dialogue had dragged on. People continued to speak on and on, endlessly, each

21

one talking past one another, without capturing let alone convincing the other. A certain weariness showed on everyone's face; people sat with drooping eyelids. Finally, Freud himself takes the floor and with one stroke all the paralyzing fatigue goes away and all eyes fix on him. Often the professor had only to utter a single sentence and the whole, endless, fruitless debate would be instantly elucidated. As Max Kahane once aptly said, "Roma locuta est, causa finita" [Rome has spoken, the case is closed]. However, this came about not because of the force of decreed infallibility but rather because each one of the listeners felt "Here was the right solution." Some people came every Wednesday just for the sake of one such single sentence that they then carried home as if it were a treasure. In the first days, it was still the custom to write the names of all the members on little slips of paper that our secretary would then draw by lot out from the urn. Whoever was selected had to speak. If by some bad luck Professor Freud was the first to speak, that made any further discussion almost superfluous. Dr. Kahane once said to me, "Once he has spoken, no more grass can grow." Since, for better or worse, what was of principal importance had already been exhaustively stated, one could at best present only a modest addendum.

No less unerring and all-consuming was also the criticism that one on occasion had from Freud in private. Thus I remember once reading him a paper in which I believed I had discovered many new things. Freud listened to me, while pacing back and forth, smoking the whole time. When I finished, he asked, "Now do you want to hear my opinion?" And then he launched into his response and gave me, then and there, reactions to all my new discoveries which he had just heard for the first time. And what reactions they were! Every word was precisely crafted and could have been published even though sometimes demolishing my findings. Where I had believed that I had found something new, it turned out that Freud had already known this all along but simply hadn't published it. And that his words were not merely empty phrases was made clear by the fact that he had already advanced so much further than I had. With one sentence, he would lead me to a last insight which I had still not seen. One, suddenly felt very small in front of the giant. That was Sigmund Freud, the critic, on good days. But there was another Freud who would occasionally like to put forth during his bad moods opposing even his most faithful followers. Then the otherwise so generous man became petty, carping, and cranky, spewing forth isolated words and phrases. No more were there signs of progress, or speeches full of creative instructive evaluation. Only extreme discomfort remained for the injured party who would have liked to have given up completely.

And now to turn to Freud the writer, the word artist and great stylist. Even a person who never had the good fortune to hear the Professor personally will be fascinated by the very special magic of his writings. I will not compare his works with the intellectual products of other psychiatrists. It is not an absolute prerequisite of science that a great scholar must also be able to write well. To be sure, "Understanding and accurate meaning can be conveyed with little art," as Goethe maintained. However, the psychiatric literature is especially rife with unbelievable jargon, much more so in comparison with other disciplines. It no longer remains comprehensible to our medical colleagues. Their principal trick, then, consists of every two years sending out into the world some technical terms, preferably as hard to understand as possible—a true theory of emissions—and managing to muddle long-understood disease diagnostics and to pour old wine into newly labeled wineskins. In my sinful youth, I had learned about adolescent madness, better known as hebephrenia, and paranoia. Later under [Emil] Kraepelin's [1856–1926] influence, the names were changed to dementia praecox and paranoides whereby not without some mischievous pleasure, it was proposed to throw out paranoia altogether replacing it with "paraphrenia" in Kraepelin's sense of the word. On the other hand, it was readily admitted that in any nice case of dementia praecox, neither dementia nor praecocitas had to be present. So surely this was truly the most appropriate designation!

But the laurels from Miltiades to Themistocles never rested so that Bleuler invented schizophrenia or schizothymia to which Kretschmer recently added schizoid personality. This once again shows how right Fritz Reuter's [1810–1874] "Uncle Bräsig" was in saying that the poor arise from great poverty. An even prettier mess was the situation when individual symptoms of schizophrenia were involved. With the help of Latin and Greek dictionaries, new technical terms were created for each of the many symptoms, terms which without exception were so wonderfully clear that one had first to explain them to the doctor. It is still worth considering the unforeseen good luck that there were so few colleagues that spoke Sanskrit that this source for psychiatric nomenclature was little used. In any case, in psychiatry one must keep up to date and above all, read its journals. Otherwise, one has to relearn everything every two years or be left behind as someone who no longer counts.

It is worth noting that mainstream psychiatry took no notice of Freud for so long other than at most a variety of malicious remarks at a time when he made an effort to use faultless German using only the simplest expressions intelligible to all. It was only during his last years when the Professor moved a little towards metaphysics—approximately after *Beyond the Pleasure Principle* [1920], and though it was not jargon, there were expressions such as Eros and Thanatos, the Ego, the Ego Ideal, and the Id, and occasionally losing himself in speculation—that Freud became more sympathetic to psychiatry. He began gradually to rise to the pinnacle of the psychiatric profession, worthy of becoming the most profound of all sciences. Now Goethe said:

> A fellow who speculates
> Is like an animal on dry heather,
> Who is led around in a circle by an evil spirit
> And all around lies beautiful green pasture.

But in the dark times of Goethe, classic psychiatry as we know it today did not yet exist.

But let us return to Freud the stylist and to the specifics of his writing style. In order to stay, first of all, with outward appearances, I would like to say that in his diction, in his sentences, everything is simple, straightforward and great. And the shorter the piece, the more delightful it is. His short papers that at the outside scarcely come to no more than eight to ten printed pages are, frankly, showcase pieces for the art of scientific presentation. Nevertheless Freud always remains a person with a great natural modesty, never forgetting that a genius is never more than a fallible human.

In one of his latest works, written whilst already surrounded by the specter of death, I read, deeply moved, these words:

"In the following pages I bring forward some findings of analytic research which would be of great importance if they could be proved to apply universally. Why do I not postpone publication of them until further experience has given me the necessary proof, if such proof is obtainable? Because the conditions under which I work have undergone a change, with implications which I cannot disguise. Formerly, I was not one of those who are unable to hold back what seems to be a new discovery until it has been either confirmed or corrected. My *Interpretation of Dreams* and my 'Fragment of an Analysis of a Case of Hysteria' [1905] were suppressed by me—if not for the nine years enjoined by Horace—at all events for four or five years before I allowed them to be published. But in those days I had unlimited time before me—'oceans of time' as an amiable author puts it—and material poured in upon me in such quantities that fresh experiences were hardly to be escaped. Moreover, I was the only worker in a new field, so that my reticence involved no danger to myself and no loss to others.

"But now everything has changed. The time before me is limited. The whole of it is no longer spent in working, so that my opportunities for making fresh observations are not so numerous. If I think I see something new, I am uncertain whether I can wait for it to be confirmed. And further, everything that is to be seen upon the surface has already been exhausted; what remains has to be slowly and laboriously dragged up from the depths. Finally, I am no longer alone. An eager crowd of fellow-workers is ready to make use of what is unfinished or doubtful, and I can leave to them that part of the work which I should otherwise have done myself. On this occasion, therefore, I feel justified in publishing something which stands in urgent need of confirmation before its value or lack of value can be decided." ["Some Psychological Consequences of the Anatomical Distinction between the Sexes," 1925]

Here in a short specimen, we find everything that makes Freud's personally painted communications so captivating: a plain, purely human narrative, full of discretion and tremendous intelligence. If the materials required it, Freud could become half poet, but he was always entirely a man of science with a nearly inexhaustible abundance of new thoughts. Sometimes these would pour out in such profusion that he could hardly manage to control them. Then the reader would have the greatest difficulty in biting through this mountain of milk and honey, and he would have to study again and again in order to scoop out everything that had been squeezed into a few lines. But this held only occasionally for what was fixed in writing, for the reading of what was printed, because in his live lectures, Freud always had compassion for his listeners and their troublesome lagging comprehension. For that reason, one can say of him as was said about Goethe: "What he spoke was better than what he wrote."

When I look over Freud's works, it seems to me that in terms of purely stylistic features, extraordinary progress is unmistakable. One remembers, for example, that his first psychoanalytic writings were certainly tentative experiments. Everything was still amply stuffed with foreign and technical terms from the witches' brew of psychiatry. Only the few case histories which so grace the *Studies on Hysteria* [1895] betray already the claw of a lion with its nearly poetic narrative talent that can transform casuistry into short stories. Then came in the first place, the great *Interpretation of Dreams* [1900] that brought new ground-breaking explanations for what was up until then as good as an incomprehensible domain of the mind. And yet how unpedagogical are his ideas almost suffocating in their enormous quantity. Five years later followed the already classically written *Three Essays on the Theory of Sexuality* [1905], in every respect totally great Freud. But even here there are several lapses into the unpedagogical. And the most widely circulated of his writings, *The Psychopathology of Everyday Life* [1901], was not free of it either where psychopathology, a proper psychiatric term, was noticeably replaced in the *Lectures* by the German word "Fehlleistung" [a failed effort or mistake]. I won't even mention some of Freud's last treatises, such as *Beyond the Pleasure Principle* [1920] and *The Ego and the Id* [1923]. At the same time, however, such works as *Delusions and Dreams in Jensen's* Gradiva [1907], *Group Psychology and the Analysis of the Ego* [1921], the classic *Introductory Lectures on Psychoanalysis* [1916–1917], as well as, finally, *The Question of Lay Analysis* [1926] are stylistic masterpieces regardless of whether or not one might raise pertinent objections to their conclusions. In truth, one cannot express enough regret that Freud was prevented from presenting the full extent of his ideas. This was because illness and advancing old age prevented him from concentrating sufficiently on permanently setting down these ideas in writing. I have just touched on a point of decisive importance with respect to Freud's particular specific genius: the abundance and correctness of his ideas. They were so overpowering due to the boldness and magnitude of his thought, the breadth of his vision, and the lightning-like penetrating connections. And then, time and time again, there was the reflective judgment as to whether there was possibly a mistake or a contradiction. Such prudence is entirely unheard of among university professors in establishing new tenets and basic principles. This is most evident in the first two parts of his *Lectures*. Freud never forces the facts to fit his theory, but always remains objective and perspicacious. And as for negative virtues, he had no trace of moral hypocrisy, he never played judge which in matters of sexuality and decency is not always an easy thing. Perhaps one will admire his objectivity even more when one finds out that Freud was at heart an awful sadist who had to force himself to be scientifically dispassionate, that further he was misunderstood for many years by his opponents, one could say often intentionally, and that finally he had the ability to destroy someone with one sentence, friend as well as foe.

So I can at this point conclusively declare: I know of no other medical researcher whose lectures and writings so impress me as being classic: simple and great.

Contributions to the Study of Freud's Character

One trait, especially, comes to the fore in a portrait of Freud's character: his incredible love of truth. To be sure, one would think that this would go without saying for any scientist. For without absolute honesty, one can not accomplish anything worthwhile in science. As a matter of fact, however, the courage to be truthful, and not be held back by one's own ego, is a great rarity, at least among mentally healthy individuals. With Sigmund Freud, there is honesty, if it becomes necessary, to the point of unsparing self-revelation. In his preface to *The Interpretation of Dreams,* he said it this way:

> "The only dreams open to my choice were my own and those of my patients undergoing psychoanalytic treatment. But I was precluded from using the latter material by the fact that in this case the dream-processes were subject to an

undesirable complication owing to the added presence of neurotic features. But if I was to report my own dreams, it inevitably followed that I should have to reveal to the public gaze more of the intimacies of my mental life than I liked, or than is normally necessary for any writer who is a man of science and not a poet. Such was the painful but unavoidable necessity; and I have submitted to it rather than totally abandon the possibility of giving the evidence for my psychological findings." [Preface to the First Edition, 1900]

Only in one point did Freud deviate from the truth, even though it was completely unconscious and stemming from his own unresolved complexes. I had to witness how he once offered Jung, who was at that time one of his pets, a discovery that he himself had made. He had simply identified himself with Jung. Naturally, this caused considerable head-shaking among the intimates of the circle and one of them made the Professor aware of the fact that the supposed discovery of Jung was already to be found in the *Three Essays on the Theory of Sexuality*. This Freud had completely forgotten and he was quite astonished when he was shown the passage in his book. This ungrudging surrender of his own thoughts will continue to concern us.

Here I would just like to mention another character trait of Freud. He had an appetite for new people, always needing other individuals who, when he was finished with them, he would, of course, get rid of with the same ease with which he had acquired them. It is really amazing how many teachers and former students Freud broke off relations with over the years after they had been so close to him for a short or long period of time. As such, I will name only the most noteworthy: Breuer and Fliess, Jung and Bleuler, Adler and Stekel, Kahane and Wittels. As is the case with severely ill mental patients, he did not allow his ego to establish any permanent or long-lasting relationships, unless such a relationship was with people who lived far away and who willingly acquiesced to everything. An old doctor once maintained, "Collegiality expands with the square of the distance." That is exactly right. From Vienna to New York, collegiality is enormously great, not much less than infinity. For England, France, and Switzerland, it is considerable. But if one lives in the same town, however, or better yet in one and the same alley, one would love to drown the beloved colleague in a glass of water.

Freud's behavior is a case in point. He got along best and for the longest time with the leaders of the groups furthest away, in London, Budapest, and Berlin. He did not come into personal contact with them very frequently; they swore blindly by his every word, and they responded to every signal that came from Berggasse (Freud's residence in Vienna). In their essays and reviews they would present literally every-thing the master desired. So they received the warm rays of the merciful sun, repaying the debt on their part with the most extreme devotion.

Freud was different in the narrower circle that came together weekly or later biweekly. To be sure, the re-cruit, the newcomer, mostly got to play first fiddle in heaven. As a rule, Freud was full of captivating amiabil-ity on those occasions, a regular "fisher of souls" as Adler once called him. No one could resist the magic of this master and he could literally win over anyone that he wished to. Then the honeymoon would be over, and one day, perhaps at a lecture where the newcomer had done his best, he had to live through the experience whereby the Professor would, so to speak, "tear him to pieces in public." Freud had the same ability to give high praise as he otherwise did to destroy and grind someone into the ground. About this, everyone in the circle had such a story to tell. For Freud deep down inside was a terrible sadist which cost his enemies less than his students and most loyal followers. None of those who stood near him or were allowed to approach him would be spared the boot, sooner or later. One person would leave him with simpering masochistic happiness; another would clench his fist in his pocket; a third preferred years of silence in order to avoid any occasion that would necessarily have led to an estrange-ment. Ever since one of the acquiescent, "the right hand of psychoanalysis" [presumably Otto Rank], quite literally a creation of Freud, living in thrall, had to learn that the path from power to the gallows is only a short distance, I was absolutely convinced that none of the closest students would be able to remain in a trouble-free harmonious relationship with the Professor for a lifetime. For the Berlin Congress [1922], the Psychoanalytic Press published an elegant bound calendar, graced with the latest photograph of Freud. When I caught sight of it, I was horrified. How could anyone have chosen such an image! That was surely the face of an ill-natured sadist, not the thinker we all knew! On the other hand, we have just this sadism as a reaction to Freud's captivating amiability to thank as characteristic consequences of his enormous energy that allowed him to oppose a world of enemies.

In the last chapter I emphasized what a superabundance of new ideas Freud constantly produced. If one had not seen him for two months, perhaps during vacation time, he was already a totally different person in conversation. One had just barely become acquainted with his last train of thought only to find out that the master was already again ten miles ahead of everyone so that keeping pace with him or catching up with him seemed impossible. Never have I had the impression of standing before another such man, before a genius, as with Freud. If the term "ingenious" applies to any mortal, not in the trivial sense, but literally, then it would apply to the Professor. He was ruled often by such an overwhelming wealth of new ideas that he alone was not able to carry them all through to completion. He had to give them away as presents in order not to be smothered by his own gold. He was a grand-master of thought who gave away ideas with princely generosity, ideas so great that a well established privy councilor and university professor could have given lectures on them for a whole semester, bringing fame and fortune to his faculty.

For years, Wilhelm Stekel had the reputation of being a bright or even a genius writer from devouring the countless ideas that Freud would toss carelessly under the table every Wednesday. What he would write in various newspapers was truly often of genius quality, but it was never a question of the genius of a Stekel, a man who with his eyes wide open could hardly discover anything, but the genius of a Freud. To be sure, this fact was not infrequently obscured in journalistic reproduction, especially since the Professor on one Wednesday evening expressly declared: "What I say here is for the taking; you can do with it as you please."

How incredibly generous Freud was with new ideas! How many of his students did he not only stimulate with such ideas—that would be self-evident and completely legitimate—but he also gave them away as a direct gift, that is to say, he not only elucidated ideas for them, but he of his own accord ceded his intellectual property, what he alone had discovered. When, generally speaking, a joint project is published, say by Privy Councilor and Professor X and Dr. Y, one could usually swear that Professor X simply provided his name in this case and "kindly," as the lovely phrase goes, "made available the material from his clinic." Everything else, however, all the real work was done by Dr. Y alone. With Freud, it was the opposite. The idea was his, and so was the astute observation, as well as the broad connections. It was merely often just the feeble execution that was left for others. If Freud, however, was full of good will, then he would take the essay of a student and improve it from beginning to end, so that the only thing remaining from the student's original contribution were the auxiliary verbs. Everything else was the Professor's contribution, only that he would then, in addition, not put his name on it and give the whole thing to his colleague as a present. At most, he would betray his collaboration by warmly defending the one under attack if an objection was raised in discussion.

The very best ideas Freud gave only rarely to local colleagues, at most just to the house factotum [Otto] Rank. Usually, chairmen of the foreign regional groups were chosen who thereby were given fame and reputation—naturally apart from their own obvious intellectual greatness. And again I am reminded of the nice phrase: "Collegiality expands with the square of the distance." Of course, one must in fairness admit that other factors played a part in the Professor's negative attitude. Above all, the extreme decisive actions of Viennese colleagues, especially the circle of experts. Did not the Viennese neurologists not only fail to recognize him, but they also ridiculed him and branded his teachings as quackery? Even those doctors who did not aspire to an academic career and thus did not have to pay attention to any puff of wind coming from above, did not they too learn that psychoanalysis was humbug, if not to say filthiness? But, as is well known, the actual validation of criticism is the very least little thing. So Freud's hostility towards the Viennese doctors is easily understood, but certainly the most innocent, especially the closest students, suffered the most. And it is possible to imagine that Freud, by favoring lay analysis, wanted to prove to his Viennese colleagues that one could by developing his talent be a first-rate psychoanalyst without necessarily having studied official psychiatry and neurology.

I have mentioned above that Freud repeatedly presented significant thoughts to selected students. In contrast to that, he was not pleased if one of them insisted that he wanted to discover something on his own. Then he would become grumpy, yes, even angry. And to be sure, not merely if the persons completely distanced themselves from him as did Adler and Jung, but also when someone like Stekel tried to set himself up as an equal to the Professor on the basis of his own little discovery. Even those who worked only with Freud's ideas and disavowed their own individuality, were looked askance at if they so much as once changed or added one little brick to the edifice.

In the most benign cases, where something really new had been discovered, the Professor listened in silence without approval. If a student, however, had missed the mark, this attempt at unauthorized individual research could lead to a break. For Freud was not merely the father of psychoanalysis, but also its tyrant! This might help explain why he did not leave behind a proper "school" even though so many stood on his shoulders and put his ideas to use. Certainly it was not easy to exist at Freud's side and even less so when he meant well. He smothered everyone with the force and greatness of his genius and those who stood closest to his emanations could not keep their limbs unscathed any more than could the first researchers of radium and x-rays. No one could really hold one's own next to this giant and many who were too weak to simply love him for what he was therefore became his enemy!

Above I spoke of Freud's modesty in all scientific things, and can add only that he always refused officially and publicly to play the leader. He presided over the first congress in Salzburg only after Bleuler had refused the chairmanship offered him. Otherwise Freud always promoted others and would always make one of his favorites President of the International Psychoanalytic

Association. To all appearances, he wanted nothing more than to be merely the chairman of a regional group, at least in name. But in truth, all the strings were held together in his firm hand and none of the others, not even the international president, would have dared to decree anything without first asking Freud. Not once did an article appear in our journal if he was not completely in accord, or if he, at the very least, did not indulgently allow it. Even when death had already stretched out his hand towards him and Freud could no longer even fulfill the duties of the chairman of the Vienna regional group, he still remained the ruler of all, the "primal father" or "Father of All" as he was still called at the Berlin psychoanalytic congress.

In *Group Psychology and the Analysis of the Ego* [1921], Freud sketched the face of a leader—modeled after himself. And he was so beloved by all in the circle of intimates and at congresses that it sparked envy among his followers. Already during the time of Adler and Stekel in the Vienna regional group, where the talents of those who stood closest to the central sun chiefly developed, there were always intense fights and jealousies. There Freud's sadism as well as his enormous genius would come to light full force.

In "On the History of the Psychoanalytic Movement," Freud also talks about the earliest meetings of the small group of disciples in his house and observes the following:

"There were only two inauspicious circumstances which at last estranged me inwardly from the group. I could not succeed in establishing among its members the friendly relations that ought to obtain between men who are all engaged upon the same difficult work; nor was I able to stifle the disputes about priority for which there were so many opportunities under these conditions of work in common."

The second point seems to me to be of less importance because the decisive, most important discoveries were made by the professor himself as everyone readily acknowledged. On the other hand, a mutually friendly state of understanding did not exist among us all—only I must say not entirely without blame on Sigmund Freud's part. He could very well have kept a tight rein on the students, if he had from the beginning of the group used his absolute authority to make crucial interventions—had he not himself, on occasion, presented a bad example to the others. How could he press for courteous friendliness and halt every attack that was not purely factual if he himself blithely disregarded both rules and to be sure, did so more than once. Understandably, since Freud could not for various weighty reasons show his displeasure to his opponents, he might on occasion let it break out against his own followers, against students and disciples. He had his moods and unpredictable temper. While his favorites were often allowed for the most part to do whatever they pleased, a lightning bolt could suddenly come out of the blue and seriously injure even the most loyal. If, however, Freud let loose his sadism, then he could not restrain the others from being "parliamentary," and attacking each other.

To stay on course with the truth, it has to be said that Freud was not free from moods, yes, one could even say that now and then he had the mood of a hysterical woman. Then he would become completely unpredictable. I will cite just two examples. I believe it was in the year 1908 that we members were suddenly surprised by a notice from the secretary of the society, Otto Rank: Freud had decided that the Society that at that time still met at his home would be dissolved in order that it could then be reconstituted anew. One was supposed to declare in writing whether or not one wished to join the new society. And what was the meaning of this otherwise entirely incomprehensible maneuver? As it soon turned out, what was planned was to get rid of Dr. Kahane for as the Professor rightly assumed, he would not make a new affiliation request. Here it is particularly worth observing that Freud owed great thanks to this sagacious, deserving, and highly respected colleague. Had he not stood up for the Professor at a time when it was plainly compromising for him to repeatedly defend his manhood. But gratitude was never Freud's strength. Kahane's crime was just that he had known the great man while he was still a little secondary school student, that is to say, while still in his tattered boots.

One day, in later years, when the Society was already meeting in its own place, Freud, all of a sudden, without any apparent motive, resigned his chairmanship, and proposed Adler in his stead with Wilhelm Stekel as deputy. After this interregnum had lasted for a few months, Freud declared just as suddenly that he was ready "because of a unanimous request" to again assume the chairmanship.

To conclude, I want to mention one more significant point. It is known that when one has been a professor for too long or has even become a privy councilor, one is usually already a half idiot. Customarily when this happens, students call a professor a "senex," that is, an old man with half a mind. But Freud, however, was never, not even in his very last years, ever disrespectfully called "senex." When could anyone have come to the conclusion that this constantly thought-generating genius had become senile. Though Freud certainly grew old and became severely damaged physically by illness and a long-lasting bodily infirmity, he always remained, intellectually speaking, a hero who could slay any opponent with one single tap of his paw.

Freud as Leader and Organizer

Among all the innate talents that Freud exercised, his organizational ability was not the very least. In the first chapter, I have told how insignificant the beginnings of this genius had been and how difficult it had been to drum up the minimal audience of three listeners for his lectures. If one compares that with today's International Psychoanalytic Association with its extension from the Netherlands to Calcutta, from Baltimore to London and Moscow, then one can respect this progress.

If Freud witnessed his triumph over his opponents still in his lifetime and was not misunderstood, neglected, or even locked up in an insane asylum as other ground-breaking geniuses such as Robert Mayer [1814–1878] and Ignaz Semmelweiss [1818–1865] were, so he could give thanks essentially to his gift of winning over people and welding them together into solid units. This was all the more necessary as he had to overcome much greater difficulties than any and all other researchers. Every genius with revolutionary new ideas must first of all conquer the masses' laziness and disinclination to think. That state of affairs is a matter of course for all geniuses. In addition, Freud also found a specific psychoanalytic resistance.

It is amazing how strong and widespread people's sexual shyness is, brought to the world through Christianity. The peoples of the Orient with their age-old culture, the classical nations of antiquity, the Greeks and the Romans, did not know such shyness. They were sensually joyful and natural. Only Christianity labeled woman as the vessel of sin and even the most natural act of sexual intercourse was an act that had to hide from the light of day. Nothing is more telling than the fact that in everyday speech the terms "sexual" and "immoral" are frequently held to be synonymous. One would think that the fine minds of the academy and above all, doctors for whom nothing human should be foreign, ought to be willing to turn away from this mistaken path. Well, that's a fine how-do-you-do! It is precisely the doctors who played the part of leaders of morality and became bigots, almost worse than their brothers from theology.

A psychiatric privy councilor tells the following nice little story: A sick woman who appeared to suffer from sexually-based hysteria was in a clinic and a young medical student—ah, youth is so impetuous—felt compelled to remark, "Mr. Privy Councilor, this would be a case for psychoanalysis!" Whereupon the privy councilor rebuffed him contemptuously, "Well now, if you want to be involved with such filth, then you can go ahead and do so." This, then, was the official view of the new methodology. It was seen as obscene filth dressed up as a science. On the other hand, one spoke also of a second reproof, namely that psychoanalysis was a Jewish invention, and therefore reprehensible, but liberal people did not say so openly. They just thought it and acted accordingly.

Under these circumstances, no aspiring youth were advised to turn towards this new theory. And yet Freud, from year to year, always found more followers. People were literally jostling to be a part of his circle and above all to be among his closest students. How can this puzzle be explained? One thing was clear: the prospect of a career was not a decisive factor, nor in the earlier years was it the prospect of a lucrative practice. Other teachers held on to their students through the hope of the benefit they would give that would allow the students the possibility of becoming Assistants, Docents, and Professors. Their disciples went into psychiatry, not because they felt an inner calling for this discipline—I would just once like to see a prodigy who felt such a calling—but rather because one could become an assistant within a half a year instead of waiting the usual period of four to six years in the clinics of an internist or surgeon. None of these considerations applied in Freud's case. Whoever attached himself to Freud abandoned from the outset any academic career and indeed any good will and respect from his colleagues. Such a student would find himself persecuted by the clinic, seen as a charlatan by doctors, and with a psychoanalytic practice progressing poorly if at all. There must have been a stronger magnetism at work to generate such pure idealism and to give up the fleshpots of Egypt and any monetary or substantial advantage.

This wonderful attraction was the result of the enormous richness of deep thoughts that Freud gave away weekly to his students in addition to what he made accessible in writings and lectures. Thus, above all, it was knowledge-starved youth that streamed towards the master, for no other clinical instructor could rival these treasures. And with him, they found what they could hear at no other clinic, from no other lectern, clearly intelligible, profoundly perceptive, in a word, depth-psychology. In the face of depth-psychology, everything that had heretofore been so-called psychiatry shriveled up. Finally young doctors and neurologists had something at hand that they had up to then searched for entirely in vain: the means of actually curing the so terribly widespread psychoneuroses.

But all this does not, however, explain how Freud could prevail in his lifetime, prevail against the resistance of clinical monopolies and the medical majority.

At best, his genius would have been sufficient to have had his statue placed in the great hall of the university after his death, when he had become harmless. How did he manage to live to see himself famous—even if without a statue?

Once again, his great intelligence and his ability to organize helped him. He did not limit himself to Austria and Germany or even to Vienna which was so hostile to him. If a prophet is nothing in his own country, then it was even more so for a revolutionary with such ideas as Freud. Thus he thought of foreign countries from the beginning: "Flectere, si nequeo superos, Acheronta movebo" stands at the top of one of his first works [If I can't change the gods, I will move Acheron (river of Hades), Virgil's *Aeneid,* Book 7, chosen by Freud as the title page epigraph for *The Interpretation of Dreams*]. Chance came to the aid of the afflicted. In Zurich, after [Auguste] Forel's [1848–1931] departure, a newer, fresher spirit arose and Eugen Bleuler was the first clinician to verify the "Freudian mechanism" at his institute. From that soon grew personal relationships leading to the psychoanalytic congresses, the "Schriften zur angewandten Seelenkunde," the founding of the "Jahrbücher" [yearbooks], as well as finally to the momentous lectures of Freud and Jung in America. Now psychoanalysis spread even further going with Jones to Canada and England, with Ferenczi to Hungary, and found enthusiastic supporters in France, Holland, and

Sweden, and in the end finally forced even the reluctant German clinics to consider it.

As the number of members of individual regional groups increased from year to year, this led to founding of two journals *(Zentralblatt für Psychoanalyse,* later continued as the *Internationale Zeitschrift für ärztliche Psychoanalyse* as well as *Imago)* and finally the Internationaler psychoanalytischer Verlag led to ever new problems for the young discipline to consider. Today, one can certainly say that there is no area in human culture that has not been illuminated and stimulated by our method, even more than Darwinism did during its heyday.

All strings, nevertheless, eventually came together in the hand of the master who alone knew how to organize everything, even when he was physically a broken man. Only those who knew Freud in his brightest period could appreciate the organizational energy that came out of his head. How he could understand someone after hearing only half a thought, how to handle each person on his own terms, how he knew how to get to the kernel of each problem in no time, and how he was able to articulate something decisive in one sentence. I remember, for example, a little talk that Jones gave as a guest as a contribution to our discussions. Since half of the Society's members understood no English, one of the experts—who was also a sharp-witted lawyer—was entrusted with the task of translating

Jones' words for the others. He tried, painstakingly enough, to adhere to the sentences and expressions of the speaker, translating them literally or providing superfluous elements, in any event, not exactly succeeding. Then finally the Professor's patience ran out, and with one angry "But no, my dear colleague! Jones meant to say such and such," he was able to explain in one single pithy sentence what neither the guest nor his translator were able to get across to the audience.

If a disciple arranged his thoughts such that an angel of the Lord couldn't fathom them and he presented undigested material to the master, the latter, often with a single word, would remove any uncertainty, and bring the partial thought to completion, thereby suddenly elevating the student so that at once he stood amazed to see how smart he had been. What a deep knowledge of humanity Freud always demonstrated when he wanted to win over a new follower! How fascinating he could be, just like another charmer and awful sadist, namely, Otto von Bismarck [1815–1898]! I recall a lecture somewhere around the year 1910. Once again, a psychoanalytic infant had discovered the Oedipus Complex on his own and hastened to present this information with the light of understanding shining in his eyes. Another teacher in Freud's place might have said something like, "Dear sir, I have known about that for fifteen years and it already appears in my *Interpretation of Dreams*." But instead

Freud kindly exclaimed, "Very remarkable! Really very remarkable!" thereby winning over the student for life. Another student once came to the Professor with the declaration that he wanted to practice psychoanalysis in order to help mankind and he received, to his amazement, the answer: "You want to help? Then you are a truly bad sadist!" The Professor had quickly realized that only a person who had repressed his own sadism would feel compelled in later years to want to help. And perhaps this is something he had learned from his own personal experience.

Speaking of the knowledge of humanity, I have never met anyone who could see through people as quickly and fully as Sigmund Freud. A younger colleague had asked the Professor for a consultation about a morphine addict who demanded an injection of an unbelievably high dose. When both doctors withdrew to confer, Freud declared, "My dear colleague, the wife is a hussy! There is nothing to be done!" "But Professor," the young doctor protested, "The wife looks after her husband day and night. I have observed this for weeks and weeks." "The wife is a hussy." So the consultation remained without result and the patient remained in the same condition. Six months later, the gem of a wife ran away from her husband with another man and eight days thereafter the morphine addict was cured.

When Bleuler began corresponding years ago with Freud, still unknown to him personally, there was a characteristic of the Zurich psychiatrist that surprised Freud very much. Freud knew very soon and very precisely what each person was about and if he sometimes occasionally made a mistake in the assessment of his surroundings, there were other factors at play: albeit his hatred of the academy and the environment of increasing self-confidence which greedily drank up the scanty praise. So it could happen from time to time, that even nonentities were allowed a certain influence though this for the most part did not last long and besides was always regulated by Freud.

Freud was truly a born leader and in his discipline, probably the only one. This was clearest when, because of illness, he had to turn over the personal leadership of the Viennese chapter to a vice president. Since he held the meetings of the executive board in his home from which the decisive directives came, it appeared that superficially little had changed. The current "Vice" would occupy the chair at the head of the room and with more or less grace give the floor to the speakers, instruct or scold the followers, and sometimes display the yearnings of dictatorship. In short, he would act as though he were actually the president. Only if it were a matter of settling a dispute with one sentence, or in clarifying a controversial question with the help of considerable experience or innate genius, then the dictator usually failed miserably. It was considered a godsend if he did not exacerbate the existing confusion.

One can boldly claim that the essential excitement of the psychoanalytic movement stemmed entirely from Freud himself. I will say nothing of the beginnings and the early years when all the foundations first had to be created by him. But also during the later times, beginning somewhere around 1914, there was not one great idea that did not directly or indirectly originate from Freud. I would mention narcissism as the most important and later the whole idea of ego-psychology stemming from unconscious guilt feelings, his last truly great discovery, to the death instinct, and the relationship between ego and id. Where Freud could not be directly influential as in the Viennese Psychoanalytic Society, he could often decisively influence the thoughts of the recipients of his longer letters. And when I read an essay that claimed to be composed in response to an oral or written stimulus of the Professor, I knew in an instant without a doubt whose brainchild lay before me. Through the force of his ideas, Freud had the leadership of the regional groups in his hands so that they most willingly modeled their views after his. How did Bismarck once put it: "My ambassadors must line up at attention upon command just like non-commissioned officers." Even among the psychoanalytic sergeants, I know of not one that did not do so. And not one dared to make a decision of importance on his own without Freud's consent or at the very least his indulgence. And here again the similarity to Bismarck catches the eye.

I have already mentioned that Freud was not pleased when a student went his own way or followed up his own thoughts independently. If such an event occurred, then an unspoken objection within him held sway: There should be no other person except me to seek and find something new. The sad experiences Freud had with Jung and Adler explain a lot, if not everything. Freud was not free of envy of his most talented disciples, if they even once found something new. He, abounding in insights, upon whose shoulders everyone admittedly stood, had the very least to fear from fellow workers. Perhaps another person would have publicly promoted his disciples. But Freud, however, was rightly aware that he was still the best one to hold the strings of his science and wanted to remain alone in control, if not always in name, then forever in reality. Here his facility for organization killed his future school at its root. When Freud departs from this earth, he leaves behind, to be sure, disciples who continue to grow further, but no one to continue his teaching.

Two factors in particular often gravely impaired Freud's profound understanding of humanity, his unerring judgment, and therewith the fruits of his organizational talents: his strong narcissism that required loudly articulated admiration and a perpetual need for favorite students. Now frankincense, as is well known, is the most deadly poison, but that can't be held against it. And that Freud who was earlier so terribly misjudged that he longed for well-deserved praise cannot be held against him either. It was not enough for him for praise to be given; it rather had to be constant and loudly stated. Whoever expressed his admiration only occasionally or betrayed it merely through their actions were continually in danger of falling out of grace. Freud sometimes reminded me of a man celebrating a jubilee who was at a banquet in his honor. When the master of ceremonies said, "It might be very embarrassing for the honored guest to be praised and admired this much that he would become dizzy," the latter responded this: "Oh, you have no idea how much praise I can endure!" If one grabbed hold of Freud through his narcissism, it would be possible, at least for very short time, to have him for oneself. But whoever was not able to flatter him—Freud called it "telling kindnesses"—had failed from the very start.

The topic of favorite students deserves its own chapter. Freud always needed one such on whom he could heap all honors, whether he was named Alfred Adler or C. G. Jung or Otto Rank. I can be most precise about the case of Adler. I am not quite sure what it was about this one that Freud so especially liked— certainly not his psychoanalytic knowledge or competence. When Jung visited Vienna for the first time and attended a meeting of our Society [March 7, 1907], Alfred Adler was chosen as the show-horse so to speak to parade in front of him. He had chosen as a topic a case of compulsive neurosis which he used as proof of the inferiority of sexual organs, masculine protest and the like. In the discussion that followed, I immediately declared that Adler's presentation had been anything but psychoanalytic. But at that time Freud was not yet ready to accept the truth and for a long time he held fast to the illusion that Adler was a psychoanalyst.

And this was typical. So long as the master was infatuated with a student, he not only remained blind to the student's shortcomings, but he also forced everyone to see the student with the same blindness. It was only many years later when he had fully broken with the favorite that he spontaneously declared that Alfred Adler had never understood psychoanalysis or practiced it.

Meanwhile, however, Adler took advantage of the favor of the Professor to increase his own personal following in the Society. More and more, most of those accepted were non-doctors but were, however, [Communist] Party members and what was even worse, they spoke only their own specific Adlerian jargon and did not act as if they were members of the Psychoanalytic Society. And they spoke and acted as though they were hosts of the house and that there was only one master: Alfred Adler. They merely bandied his catch phrases around and a stranger would never have suspected that Freud's teachings were being promulgated. The bubble burst when Adler finally founded a second competing society for himself and his friends but without giving up membership in the Viennese Psychoanalytic Society.

A motion, clearly with Freud's consent, was made and adopted that declared such "ambivalence" unacceptable. Adler and his group resigned and founded a "Society for Free Psychoanalysis" thus a "lucus a non lucendo" [a grove from not being full of light], a psychoanalysis that was devoid of Freud. Only later when the society was more honestly re-named as the "Society for Individual Psychology" could nothing be said against it any longer. According to a joke of one of our colleagues, everyone was free to also become a member of an animal protection society. But how important Adler and his students still find the popular term "psychoanalysis" today may be illuminated by the fact that when short advertisements about Adler's successes in France and America appear in the newspapers, the designation "the psychoanalyst" Adler was always used.

Also in the case of Jung did Freud wait until the last minute to cut the cord between himself and his favorite. It speaks not less for the truth of psychoanalysis and for the organizational talent of its discoverer that after the break had been completed, nearly all the students in both hemispheres joined Freud and not Jung. Even those whom Jung had personally introduced to psychoanalysis such as parson [Oskar] Pfister [1873–1956] remained true to the old flag. Also the Swiss regional group held firm to the Freudian tradition, to say nothing of all the rest.

Freud and the Clinic

Motto:
"Fortunate is the man who feels foreign greatness
And who makes it his own through love.
For to be great is granted to few,
And he who closes his heart to foreign appreciation,
Lives alone in a desolate self,
A sufferer—certainly a common one."

Grillparzer

Seldom is a scientific genius so often played false as was Sigmund Freud. At a banquet in his honor, years ago, I made the following speech: "If a new doctrine arises in medicine which is not begotten by a clinician, it will run through three stages, assuming that it will ultimately prevail. In the first phase, the most dangerous one, the new discipline is hushed up. In the second, it is reviled. If it nevertheless persists despite all the hostility, then one day a learned scholar will reveal that in essence the study says nothing new, but on the contrary that Hippocrates, who, as we know, knew everything, at the very least, already anticipated this study. Freud's discoveries were as good as silenced for at least a decade. They are now still in the phase of being reviled. But I personally hope to live to see them discussed so naturally as if they were already known to the Greeks and Romans."

What I said in the year 1903 has since then almost become a reality. Among clinical psychiatrists, only a single one, Eugen Bleuler, found the courage for a period of time to openly speak in favor of Freud and his teachings and yes—horribile dictu—even say so in print. Two years later, he, the discoverer of "ambivalence" found his way back, to be sure, to mainstream psychiatry and explained at the congress in Breslau in his "Critique of Freudian Theory" (*Allgemeine Zeitschrift für Psychiatrie,* vol. 70, p. 665): "My earlier discussion predominantly emphasized the positive. This present work provides a supplement to it and must 'naturally' stress more strongly the negative." This happened despite the fact that as an honest man, he had confessed that he had "no basis for modifying even in the smallest detail anything he had assumed two years earlier." How did Schmock put it in [Gustav] Freytag's *Die Journalisten*? "I have written left and right; I can write in any direction." Nowadays, he would have doubtless maintained that he was simply being ambivalent. Also Bleuler's student, C. G. Jung, to whom I will return later, went down a similar path. In modern times academic psychiatry has begun to absorb Freud's teachings, not officially but at the perineal lymph tract. It was readily accepted at home, but not yet under the linden trees.

In general, a person in the clinic is resistant to new teachings unless they are revealed by a supreme deity himself or a scholar well versed in those new teachings. Usually, the ones in authority are frightened of the *homo novus:* "He thinks too much. Such men are dangerous" [Shakespeare's *Julius Caesar,* I, ii]. Thus anyone seeking an academic career is strongly advised: "Watch out for too much intellect and talent!" And to complete that thought: whoever has genius at his disposal must conceal it with great care as it is something that the reigning privy councilor himself does not usually possess. And where would university activities end up if only proclaimed geniuses were hired, especially those who did not have eighteen Christian ancestors on both the father's and mother's side?

Freud flouted these principles of academic hierarchy, in the most grievous way. Once years ago when there had been a particularly malicious attack on him, I responded with: "You are operating on the basis of a false assumption. Freud is not a professor, Freud is a genius! One can make a professor out of any halfway intelligent man who works for a couple of years in a clinic. And when he completes his baptism, he cannot fail to attain a position and honor. On the other hand, one is born a genius and, to be sure, the birth of such doesn't occur all that often. One can become a professor, but one must **be** a genius!"

Let us take as an example the case of Freud. When he began, he still conducted himself in a manner halfway scientific and quite conformist. He even received his docentship for a kind of school exercise. Then he committed the incredible folly of discovering a whole series of groundbreaking things.

And if that wasn't enough, he did not slack off, creating something new and unheard of, year after year. Here is not the place to recap all of his scientific achievements. But to name only a few: Freud has led us to an understanding of the nature of psychoneuroses and "last not least" [original in English] also taught us how to cure them; he stimulated psychiatry in extraordinary ways, a field that was not even his own; he showed for the first time the mechanism of dementia praecox, paranoia and paranoid conditions, melancholy, mania, and cyclic mental illness; he created a new psychology: the study of the repressed unconscious and thereby inspiring, indeed, in many ways decisively the operation of countless human sciences; he was the first to really research and fully interpret dreams—and all this without really being officially authorized to do so. How could such an intelligent man have acted in such an extremely irresponsible way!

Now, however, we can see Freud's fundamental error. All his life, he had nurtured the hope that he could win over the clinic, thereby forgetting that for people of his sort this was quite impossible. Democritus once said that ever since Pythagoras offered a hundred oxen to the gods after discovering his famous theorem, all oxen tremble whenever a new discovery is made. And now along came a genius who discovered new truths year after year. Must not all the not-so-great talents feel terribly distressed in their need to justify their existence? Where would one be if every single genius that ran by was permitted to boldly overturn everything one had so painstakingly learned with one's backside on school benches!

So let this be a warning for every aspiring student: The clinic does not allow itself to be conquered; one must be born into the clinic! A malicious mind once asserted, "In the medical faculty, genius is inherited from father to son; in the philosophy department from privy councilor to the son-in-law." That is stated so generally that it is, naturally, not true. Everyday experience does teach us that there are also sons-in-law on the medical faculty, as well as more distant brothers-in-law and other relatives with hereditary talent. One can objectively say only this: The paths along which genius is inherited remain shrouded at this time. Nevertheless— one thing is clear today—they are excluded from the limited circles of professors.

Now to return again to our case. Why wasn't Freud the son of a privy councilor? Why did he not stem from an old Austrian and self-respecting Aryan office-holding family? Why didn't he at the very least marry into a professorship as a son-in-law? How easily and effortlessly, without any expenditure of overflowing talent, could he have then accomplished his ascent! Instead of this beginning, he had the lack of foresight to come into the world as a Jew and in the bargain, bringing with him yet so much genius that a whole faculty could easily have been endowed with it.

And then he put a crown on his eccentricity and began to concern himself with sexuality which was as un-Christian as it was unscientific. Does then, in general, something like a sexual instinct exist? I mean naturally by that not the so-called respectable variety which is indispensable for the propagation of the human race, not—and here my pen is ready to resist— the reproductive drive whose results indeed also nourish church and state, but rather, pure and simple, the sex drive, its consequences and symptoms. And then Freud uncovered the fact that psychoneuroses without exception are invariably based upon repressed sexual impulses, and that such sexual factors play an enormous role in mental illnesses. That must have been the last straw! How was it that another Jewish genius, Heinrich Heine [1797–1856], once gibed:

> "Love must be Platonic,
> Said the scrawny privy councilor."

And there is nothing more chaste known on earth, nothing more morally perfect than a privy councilor of psychiatry. One can understand the fate that Freud of necessity had to encounter when he addressed the Viennese Neurological Society for the first time with his doctrine. A airless space was formed around him, he who had so boldly dared to shake the world out of its sleep. And weren't the psychiatrists exactly right when they branded such views as "Jewish-sexual nonsense"?

It is not hard to imagine the further fate of the genius. Freud stood completely alone for ten years, if one disregards the small community of students that began to gradually gather around him. His writings were simply hushed up by the technical press or at best were once condescendingly and scornfully dismissed by the pinnacle of academic knowledge. Dear God, a private docent with new ideas! For a very long time, the most sure and suitable path to a professorship was to write a book against Freud and his teachings, even if one no longer knew what these teachings were about. Why even go to the trouble of seeking out the lion in his den? One had indeed heard enough deprecatory remarks about Freud in the technical literature and from big names. A conscientious student might perhaps leaf through a little bit of Freud's oldest writing, the *Studies on the Theory of Hysteria* [1895] by Breuer and Freud, although this had already long been characterized as totally obsolete by the master himself. If such a modern Don Quixote came running to attack an abandoned fortress armed with his entire schoolroom knowledge, then he would feel himself far superior to Freud and all analysts.

Meanwhile the fame of the master extended to ever wider circles, becoming more international day by day and finally could no longer be overlooked. After the Great War, Vienna became all the more a Mecca for foreign doctors and one made a pilgrimage to Freud as one had once gone to Weimar for Goethe. Freud became the most popular man in England and America, notwithstanding King George, Lloyd George, and the respective president of the United States. And when such an American doctor set foot on Viennese soil, his first question was: "Where is Freud's clinic?" That something like a Wagner clinic existed was not something that he from the other side of the big fishpond had ever even heard of. Something serious, very serious for the medical school to ponder!

But the Lord does not abandon His own and suddenly a miracle occurred. Certainly not the kind of miracle that one can read about in sacred books and books of legends, but a miracle nonetheless. Since time immemorial there had been two chairs for psychiatry in Vienna, as there had been for surgery and internal medicine. But one day—the miracle had not announced itself through any sort of signs, the animals had not become restless and the sun had not darkened—only suddenly the second chair entirely disappeared from the surface of the earth. If you please, this is no fairytale, but an actual and true miracle, happening in the twentieth century after the birth of Christ. That by this means a monopoly was created for the first psychiatric clinic, its executive board was free from any possible disagreeable rivalry with a towering genius, openings became available for the appointment of assistants, docents and professors, as well as detaching positions from neurology—all this was certainly an unexpected but not to be undervalued consequence of the miracle.

Even more, this miracle made it possible to be generous to Freud. One does not finally want to stand in front of the afterworld as a kind of Beckmesser [Sixtus Beckmesser, the town clerk in Richard Wagner's *Die Meistersinger,* foil to the hero Walther von Stolzing] who has suppressed genius with all one's might and main. Accordingly, it was decided to confer upon Freud in addition to his previous private docentship the title of a regular Austrian University Professor. But note well, only the title, of course. And so one was surprised to read in the official Viennese newspaper that the federal president had named private docent Dr. Sigmund Freud as a regular university professor. Was this not a sign of clinical generosity and moreover it was also so harmless! The state didn't pay private docents a cent and the mere title did not entitle one to the leadership of a clinic, a true teaching forum. So everything was thus in perfect order. The Austrian Republic didn't have to go to any expense, the privy councilor retained his monopoly, and the genius received an empty title. (Freud's seventieth birthday was celebrated all over the world—with the exception of the Austrian Ministry of Education and the University of Vienna. Despite this slight, the Viennese socialist city council named him a citizen—though not an honorary citizen—a distinction that was at the same time also given to an Assistant Chairman, a choir master, and a lawyer who had similarly just turned seventy years old. One can see that the city to whose fame he had so enormously contributed knew how to honor its great son.)

Nor is this fate entirely novel. When [Franz] Grillparzer [1791–1872] retired as director of the archives after twenty-four years of service, he received in addition to his not very substantial pension the title of privy councilor. At that time, this grouch of a poet wrote the following epigram:

"The titles of my works
I have been fairly paid for;
The title after title given me
Have no financial value!"

68

Quite frankly, this analogy is not perfect. Freud's nomination to be an Austrian privy councilor is missing. Thus our genius was spared this worst degradation, this last and truly Austrian disgrace!

Yet the generosity of the clinic was not depleted by its first accommodation. It allowed—one imagines—two clinical assistants of psychiatry to join the Viennese Psychoanalytic Society, not to learn anything about psychoanalysis—my God why would a clinical assistant need to know that at all—but rather, indeed, how should I paraphrase it? Briefly, they became members of the Society, and one of them later even gave lectures on psychoanalysis—evidently at the clinic.

A fine chess move, truly worthy of the cleverness of the Vatican! After one could no longer very well really ignore psychoanalysis, attempts were made to downgrade it to the ranks of a mere auxiliary science or a method of healing, something like lumbar puncture or hypnosis. Thus it became possible to demonstrate that in the clinic, one could learn not only psychoanalysis but, in addition, other psychotherapeutic methods, including all of neurology and psychiatry! How much higher before long did the all-encompassing clinic stand in comparison with the shabby Psychoanalytic Society with its small, limited field of activity! It was studiously overlooked, so as not to make one's opponent seem even larger, that psychoanalysis is no propaedeutic auxiliary science like percussion and auscultation that one can quickly learn on the side in a course but is rather an explanatory and healing technique, the principal part of a neurological practice to treat all psychoneuroses. Nor would they let it appear that in theory it was a means of rejuvenating arteriosclerotic and calcified psychiatry. This activity reminds me of the well known humorous quip of Maier. He once bragged: "All poets are full of praise and glory in extolling the splendor of May. How beautiful and magnificent must then a 'May-er' be!" If psychoanalysis is already so great, then so much more so is the clinic which reigns over not only psychoanalysis—surely a *lucus a non lucendo*—but also everything else.

After finishing with Jupiter, it is fitting to say a word about the gods of the minor clans. A second psychoanalytic society had formed in Vienna—I am not referring to that of Adler-Platte or that of Stekel—led by an extraordinary professor and former assistant in psychiatry. This society sought to approach and be in contact with the Freudian circle and was naturally very furious when the lovingly offered hand was not grasped enthusiastically. Of course, the founders themselves and even more so their supporters had for years made fun of Freud. Now, however, they were generously ready to forget all the wrongs they had very likely committed and were ready to sit down together with those they had called names and smoke a peace-pipe. Yet how narrow-minded were once again the psychoanalysts who did not want anything to do with the proffered friendship! Did they not know the words of [Johann] Nestroy [1801–1862], "It is so noble to place one's hand in the hand of another which should have rightly been placed in his face"?

The Swiss were a whole other sort! How Bleuler without new data gradually retreated from admiring Freud back to mainstream psychiatry, I have already spoken of above. Yet more drastic was *Transformations and Symbolisms of the Libido* [1912] by C. G. Jung, his student and assistant. In his noble Siegfried role, which would certainly be a splendid leading part in any *Nibelungen* movie, he was the "enfant gâté" [spoiled brat] of psychoanalysis, the absolute darling of gods and men. Freud was ready to attribute to him all possible great qualities without verification and unhesitatingly chose to make him president of the International Psychoanalytic Society and hoped through him to be able to conquer the clinic. But he had not reckoned with Jung's Christian inheritance.

As the son of a pastor, Jung had been infected with Aryan blood from his family. Deep in his heart, he was anything but a philosemite. Now, however, he encountered Judaism in its most highly gifted embodiment and Jewish knowledge shining in front of him. Was it any wonder that he began by being blinded with the feeling that never before had he stood before the countenance of a greater genius? But his lineage was not to be denied. One day he sat down and carried out scholarly studies for months which resulted in his finding his way back through the Mithra cult to primeval Christianity. In practical terms, this may be seen that as a Christian prophet, he fully stripped the libido of its sexual character and reduced it to merely spiritual energy. This was, so to speak, the decontamination of the poisonous Freudian teachings through Christianization and total cleansing. But since the master could not easily go along with this desexualization of his teachings which went to the original foundation of his theories, he saw with a heavy heart that he needed to cut the cord between him and the clinic.

In order for us to summarize all that has been said up to now, I must say again: it is still rare that so much perfidy and mean-spiritedness has been directed, sometimes entirely in the open but even more often covertly and maliciously, against Freud, a one-of-a-kind creative genius, a veritable plant of the century. That he was able to succeed in spite of this and, to be sure, still in his lifetime, he can thank, in addition to his scientific achievements, and especially his eminent intelligence, the fact that he turned to foreign countries at just the right time. This then finally forced his fatherland to grant him some recognition even if given reluctantly.

Freud at the Psychoanalytic Congresses

Freud's portrait would be incomplete if one did not take into consideration the role which he was called upon to play at the psychoanalytic congresses. I would like to highlight four of these which remain especially vivid in my memory: the first in Salzburg; the two contentious congresses in Nuremberg and Munich, and finally the last that the Professor still attended in person, the one in Berlin in the year 1922.

For every participant the first gathering in Salzburg was unforgettable, not just because the entire core group, the whole general staff of psychoanalysis, was gathered at that time in one place. Together with all the Viennese students were the clinicians Jung, Bleuler and Otto Gross [1877–1920], plus from afar Abraham and Ferenczi, Jones and [Abraham] Brill [1874–1948]. But the greatest impression was made by the content of the scientific lectures. There weren't many of these and they were all given in one single morning. Yet at no other congress have I heard so many substantial talks. Not a single one was hollow and worthless, meaningless or mere chatter; most of them, however, stood out because of a special vision. And most memorable of all was the Professor's own talk about compulsive neurosis.

Before the congress, Freud had asked his Vienna guard not to bother him before he spoke. And with good reason, as his main concern was "today to touch the king's stone heart," in other words, to win over the Swiss and above all the ambivalent Bleuler. And then the Professor spoke initially for the short half hour that had been allotted as speaking time for all the participants. Thereupon he interrupted himself with a question to the full audience whether in the light of what he still had to say, could he continue to speak? And when his request was granted with jubilation, he spoke for another hour and fifteen minutes, thus for a total of one and three-quarters hours as he was accustomed to doing in his Saturday lectures. And how he lectured! I can still clearly see today how the Swiss became wide-eyed. This was not the ordinary professorial lecture that in essence repeated what others had said and that was, in any case, readily available in textbooks. Here they began to experience all the magic of Freudian eloquence. This time the Professor had carefully brought the sea of faces to his point of view. At another place, as I have already mentioned, when he had held forth on the same theme to the Viennese Society with a superabundance of new and overpowering thoughts, it almost suffocated the audience. But in Salzburg, everything was measuredly concentrated and organized, his many discoveries reduced to the lowest common denominator of understanding among his disciples, and yet his remarks were always full of thought, even down to the auxiliary verbs. Everyone felt that just at that moment a genius had revealed himself and when it was over, all hands clapped in spontaneous applause. Under the influence of this, even Bleuler himself did not take long to use the expressive turn of phrase: "The master of us all, Professor Freud."

And then came the time of the fervent love for C. G. Jung. At the second congress which took place in Nuremberg, the Viennese experienced a frightful surprise. Without first informing anyone, Freud had agreed with Ferenczi upon a proposal that, if it were accepted, would have put all the power in the hands of the Swiss. The leadership of the movement should then move from Vienna to Zurich, where the locus of editorial control of all general analytic articles would be established, and finally it was proposed that Jung become the permanent president. This was a full-fledged dispossession and neglect of the Vienna school in favor of Jung—at that time there wasn't even a Swiss regional group—who was to be the convenient recipient of the entire future of Freud's teachings in spite of his thus far meager experience in psychoanalysis.

In "On the History of the Psychoanalytic Movement," Freud explained the motivation for this step as follows:

"I judged that the new movement's association with Vienna was no recommendation but rather a handicap to it. A place in the heart of Europe like Zurich, where an academic teacher had opened the doors of his institution to psychoanalysis, seemed to me much more promising. I also took it that a second handicap lay in my own person, opinion about which was too much confused by the liking or hatred of the different sides. I wished therefore to withdraw into the background both myself and the city where psychoanalysis first saw the light. Moreover, I was no longer young; I saw that there was a long road ahead, and I felt oppressed by the thought that the duty of being a leader should fall to me so late in life. Yet I felt that there must be someone at the head. I knew only too well the pitfalls that lay in wait for anyone who became engaged in analysis, and hoped that many of them might be avoided if an authority could be set up who would be prepared to instruct and admonish. This position had at first been occupied by myself, owing to my fifteen years' start in experience which nothing could counterbalance. I felt the need of transferring this authority to a younger man, who would then as a matter of course take my place after my death. This man could only be C. G. Jung, since Bleuler was my contemporary in age; in favor of Jung were his exceptional talents, the contributions he had already made to psychoanalysis, his independent position and the impression of assured energy which his personality conveyed. In addition to this, he seemed ready to enter into a friendly relationship with me and **for my sake to give up certain racial prejudices which he had previously permitted himself**. I had no inkling at that time that in spite of all these advantages the choice was a most unfortunate one, that I had lighted upon a person who was **incapable of tolerating the authority of another,** but who was still less capable of wielding it himself, and whose energies were relentlessly devoted to the furtherance of his own interests." [emphasis added by Sadger]

The reasons which the Professor here alleges are in no way the only possible ones and in part are simply post-hoc rationalizations. One will be able to see this when I relate the further fate of the Freud-Ferenczi proposal. After this had taken place, there was a tremendous uproar among the Viennese, a veritable palace revolution, such that Freud could hardly have expected or feared. Feelings varied with individuals, and were at first embittered rage, then offended ambition, finally passionate rebellion that roared through everyone, leading to strong opposition to the proposal. The Vienna group was not only the largest in number but altogether the single most comprehensive one. It seemed impossible to outvote them if they remained unified.

In vain, Freud tried to persuade us: "They are all ten years ahead of us in terms of practical experience (this was the bonbon in order to win us over, given with the pretense of being reluctantly acknowledged). So long as psychoanalysis has its center in Vienna, it will always be considered a Jewish science and will never be able to conquer the clinic." But the Viennese stood firm. So Freud had to back down taking all considerations into account. What he summarized in "On the History of the Psychoanalytic Movement," is not correct:

> "Finally the Viennese 'gave in,' after having succeeded in insisting that not Zurich, but the place of the residence of the President should be the center of the Association, and that he should be elected for two years."

Had Freud wanted to propose nothing other than he wished to choose Jung to be president for two years, then there would have been no resistance at all. It was only the presidency for life, his permanent right to exercise censorship, and the longtime duration of the removal of the leadership to Zurich that had stirred up the storm of indignation. On all these points, it was Freud who had "given in," not the Viennese. (Freud's description of the events at the Nuremberg congress is just as biased as that of Stekel.) How this resistance had saved Freud's teachings from great harm would be proven after a couple of years.

The reasons that induced Freud to take these actions lay far deeper than he might have liked to admit. Already before the Nuremberg congress he had become quite ill-tempered in front of the Viennese students because of the excess of talent that they had accumulated among them. He once spoke of it directly: "With the talent that is concentrated in Vienna one could establish a dozen regional groups." And it is furthermore not surprising that students would often provoke one another, especially since the master occasionally presented a model with his hussar attacks. Instead of gently intervening, which would certainly have been very possible given his authority, Freud, shortly before Nuremberg, in a fit of pique, renounced the presidency and installed Adler and Stekel as vice-presidents. With Jung, whom he loved, he hoped to have an easier time. For the Bismarck of psychoanalysis was more concerned with real power than with semblance of same. Finally, he tried to convince himself at that time that if psychoanalysis could only be Christianized, then its Jewish origin could surely be forgiven.

But how very much mistaken Freud had been about Jung in his ability "to renounce racial prejudice," as with his compliance with the master. It became ever more clear as Jung openly proceeded with his own libido theory and as he sought to eliminate Jewish sexuality from the study of neuroses. Freud, who had long been very reluctant to recognize his favorite student's desertion, was finally compelled to cut the cord between himself and Jung so as not to permanently endanger the future of psychoanalysis. At the Munich congress, he finally resolved to pronounce the liberating words of separation: "That is your teaching, and no longer my teaching!" Almost all the regional groups went with the master, only a very few Swiss remained with Jung. And psychoanalysis cannot thank them in truth for any new blossoms. The results teach us how fruitless the Jungian modifications have proven to be during the time when psychoanalytic research under Freud's leadership has continued its triumphal course.

There is yet one additional congress that I shall briefly mention—the meeting in Berlin in September of 1922—since it was the last time that Freud spoke in a circle of all his own. The lectern had been placed for him opposite an armchair, in order to outwardly document that he was in a class by himself. Sitting in this armchair, he tirelessly listened to three days' worth of not always very exciting lectures. For a sixty-six year old who, as would soon become obvious, was no longer in good health, it was, speaking purely physically, an astonishing feat. It was frequently noted that Freud, who was not allowed to smoke in this place, while listening, always had his finger playing around in his mouth, thus again going back to the oral erotic stage of an infant. "And the great do not fear to show their needs." I have sketched in the second chapter how Freud in his own lecture on the conscious and unconscious enchanted his listeners, and above all, throwing the idea of unconscious feelings of guilt out into the crowd. This was his swan song; for many of his younger students this was their only memory of the great man and his art of lecturing.

Freud's Wit

One side of Freud's character, hardly known to the outside world, and mostly manifested only within a narrow circle, has therefore naturally been little appreciated. Yet it still appears to me to be important enough to devote an entire chapter to it. I am referring to his wittiness which only on occasion rose to the level of liberating humor. Not without reason is one of his earliest works called *Wit and Its Relation to the Unconscious* [1905], using the term "Wit" not "Humor." A sense of joy and good humor, the basis for the last, were much less present in this genius than the always sadistically tinged irony, a lightning-like satirical illumination, and even a deadly jibe. As far back as I can remember, I never heard him give a hearty, liberating, resounding laugh. At best, if a joke was suddenly right to the point, for an instant a laugh would break out, something like a cough, or Freud would distort the corner of his mouth into a scornful smirk. Perhaps this was where the countless bitter disappointments he as a great scientific revolutionary encountered were worked out. And with the passing years, these disappointments became all the more burdensome as his genius appeared more and more threatening to those in power. He repressed everything that he did not tell his enemies to their face in spite of the fact that he was perfectly capable of doing so and then put the deadly displaced emotions into his laughter making his wit sharply pointed, now and then, even having the taste of bitter gall. It seems significant to me that his favorite humorists to whom he returned again and again were Wilhelm Busch [1832–1908] and Nestroy, not, for example, Fritz Reuter [1810–1874] and Otto Ernst [Schmidt, 1862–1926].

I will try to reconstruct from my memory a couple of examples of this kind of wit. The Viennese Psychoanalytic Society had admitted a new member, a doctor of medicine and philosophy. He possessed the prized trait of being able to publish books effortlessly. In conversation, he demonstrated an often brilliant dialectic and since he did not understand all that much of psychoanalysis, he compensated for this lack through narrative eloquence. When Freud was told of a lecture on psychoanalysis that Dr. X had given elsewhere, he acknowledged it curtly: "Ah, X, the philosopher!" And about another psychiatrist, he declared, "To be an asylum psychiatrist is the mildest form of internment."

It was in Austria during the hardest time of the post-war period. The crown seemed to be sinking into a bottomless abyss, the cost of a living wage had climbed enormously, a million was so to speak like a small coin. The Austrian government, no longer able to satisfy the hunger of its civil servants, was, however, therefore all the more generous in the conferring of all kinds of empty titles. In particular, the formerly highly regarded title of privy councilor was issued in large numbers, an unjustifiable act as courts in the federal state no longer existed. About this Freud once laconically expressed his opinion: "Now the ideal of every true Austrian has been fulfilled: each is firstly a privy councilor; each is secondly a millionaire."

After Freud had been operated on for a malignant tumor and soon thereafter for a second time because of metastasis, the circle of initiates gave him at best only a year to live. The year slipped by, but the Professor made no sort of preparation to die, but rather, quite on the contrary, he began gradually to recuperate. Freud, of course, had not failed to notice the countenances of his associates, enemies as well as "friends," and after the year that had been allowed him had passed without bringing him the expected end, he said ironically, "Never have I seen so many disappointed faces!"

Once there was a conversation about a highly intelligent brain anatomist whom the bureaucracy in its wisdom had named as a professor of psychiatry. Freud had this to say about him: "The truth is that he is not knowledgeable about mental illness. However, because he is a privy councilor and a full professor, no one noticed this. For him, all of psychiatry was simply the field upon which his genius could romp."

Another time, he told a story about the same privy councilor: "I had returned from France with the news that hysteria also occurred with men. Who should provide the most strenuous opposition in the Neurological Society but this same scholar and naturally the privy councilor was held to be right—as in all such cases. However, when a few years later, he lay near death and I visited him for the last time eight days before he died, he told me, 'You were absolutely right with your contention. The very best example of masculine hysteria is—I myself.'" Moreover, this is a strikingly illuminating example of why so many of Freud's teachings stirred up such malicious, unconscious personal antagonisms.

Once Freud was invited by an academic organization to give a talk about sexual abstinence. So far as I can recall, he spoke as follows: "There is much to say about this question, both for and against. Certainly, in general, one must say that as a neurologist, I know of no cases where too much sexual activity has been harmful. Here nature herself in the case of men bars too much activity. On the other hand, however, a good many people suffer from the consequences of abstinence. And perhaps I will have the laughers in the audience on my side if I tell you a humorous story: In every family, there is some kind of aunt who asks the little children stupid questions. So one such aunt once asked an alert six-year-old boy: 'Why do we have teeth?' And she received the fresh, cheeky answer: 'To brush them.' Of course! A silly question deserves just such a smart-aleck answer. 'And why do we have sexual organs?' 'Well now, obviously for abstinence.'" I have never heard the question of sexual abstinence answered in a shorter, cleverer, and more honest way.

Among the oldest members of the intimate circle was, for a long time, a colleague who habitually made psychoanalysis understood through newspaper articles, thereby, however, pushing his own seemly greatness into the foreground. We will call him Dr. Serenus [Wilhelm Stekel]. With a very lively disposition, he would latch on to every new idea without further maturation and without the slightest qualm would call the same thing white today and black tomorrow, and indeed often exclaim, "I've always said the thing is white (or black)," depending upon his particular conviction at the time. Once, when he again came out in our circle with a profuse smattering of ideas, the Professor tersely replied: "My dear colleague, having new ideas is not what matters—they are as cheap as blackberries—but rather it matters that they are right!" Another time, with his familiar voice of deep conviction, Dr. Serenus proclaimed, "No psychoanalyst can deny that the case is such and such!" Whereupon the Professor calmly replied that he wanted only to ask Dr. Serenus whether he considered him [Freud] as a psychoanalyst since he took the liberty to say that he was of the opposite opinion as the honorable previous speaker.

Ten years had passed since the appearance of *Studies on Hysteria*. On its anniversary day, the intimates put on a small celebration. A cake had been baked on which had been written in icing "Studies on Hysteria, 2nd Edition." One of the individual organizers, in a humorous speech, explained that on the anniversary day, a new edition of the groundbreaking book had appeared, but only one single copy and, handing Freud a knife, asked the author to cut it open. Dr. Serenus, who always loved big words, interrupted in a joking manner, "Professor Freud doesn't cut open!" [doesn't brag]. Freud, however, thus provoked, then handed the knife to Dr. Serenus with the polite words: "Then, if you please, my dear colleague!"

In a dialogue, one of the disciples had spoken very profoundly such that then the master gave this verdict: "Much was spoken today and it was so clever that I have understood nothing at all." About his opponents, Freud once commented, "It is curious how otherwise very smart people suddenly become stupid when their own complexes are alluded to. Then the most threadbare arguments are now good enough for them and explanations they would otherwise dismiss with disdain appear to them suddenly noteworthy. One could call this behavior 'resistance-stupidity' or 'emotional feeble-mindedness.'" Bleuler once rightly wrote: "One cannot discuss Freudian theories in the same way as other theories one is not able to accept. One has to take affect into account as if Freud had seduced one's own wife. That is sexual repression."

True humor without any thorns is only occasionally encountered in Freud. So, for example, in the first section of the otherwise charming work "On the History of the Psychoanalytic Movement." Whoever wants to be angry at the master for that should keep in mind that he was a Jew, the greatest genius at the University of Vienna, and yet still persecuted with hostility like no other researcher. It is the literal truth when he writes:

> "Vienna has done everything possible, however, to deny her share in the origin of psychoanalysis. In no other place is the hostile indifference of the learned and educated section of the population so evident to the analyst as in Vienna."

And perhaps what the shrewd Swiss critic C. A. Loosli [1877–1959] said recently in his book *The Terrible Jews* [1927] is relevant: "The Jew has no humor; he has wit because humor is the expression of those who have overcome the softened ones. Wit, in contrast, belongs to those who are hardened, always signifying renewed suffering. It is wonderfully sharp, pointed, caustic; it is not afraid of cruel self-ridicule, this Jewish wit of which we Aryans catch only the lightning-like brilliance and enjoy but, however, are not able to recognize the narrow focal point that goes back to a reflection of corrosive suffering. We can recognize it only if we ourselves are unfortunate enough, that is, if it was the case that we ourselves were witty. He of us who is able to disclose a full understanding of the Jewish joke, the richest fruit of this wit together with its deep substratum, and its entire origins, would benefit the Jews' fraternization with us. Through such fraternization, the sources of Jewish wit would be exhausted, as that intellectuality towards which the best of mankind strives would be shared with us."

It was a minor sensation when Freud wrote a significant paper "Humor" for the psychoanalytic congress in Innsbruck [1927, the paper was read at the congress by Anna Freud]. Whoever heard this lecture at that time understood why the Professor came to the treatment of this material so late in his life. In essence, the paper merely brought humor into line with the most recent ego-theories of Freud and he could not have written it earlier because up until then, there was no such theory. Certainly what we heard here was true Freud, with insight achieved through work rich in ideas that is always peculiar to the individual scholar. The talk contained many significant and quite surprising new things. But the deepest nature of humor was not explained, perhaps just because Freud did not have any humor himself.

Freud and Judaism

"I was born on May 6th, 1856, at Freiberg in Moravia, a small town in what is now Czechoslovakia. My parents were Jews **and I too have remained a Jew**. I have reason to believe that my father's family were settled for a long time on the Rhine (at Cologne), that as a result of a persecution of the Jews during the fourteenth or fifteenth century, they fled eastwards, and that, in the course of the nineteenth century, they migrated back from Lithuania through Galicia into German Austria." [emphasis added by Sadger]

Thus reads the beginning of an autobiography that Freud wrote in 1925 for the collection *Medicine of the Present-day in Self-Portraits.* And he then continues:

"When, in 1873, I first joined the University, I experienced some appreciable disappointments.

Above all, I found that I was expected to feel myself inferior and an alien because I was a Jew. I absolutely refused to do the first of these things. I have never been able to see why I should feel ashamed of my descent or, as people were beginning to say, of my race. **I put up, without much regret, with my non-acceptance into the community;** for it seemed to me that in spite of this exclusion an active fellow-worker could not fail to find some nook or cranny in the framework of humanity. These first impressions at the university, however, had one consequence which was afterwards to prove important; for an at early age I was made familiar with the fate of being in the Opposition and of being put under the ban of the 'compact majority.' The foundations were thus laid for a certain degree of independence of judgment." [emphasis added by Sadger]

Let us now add what Sigmund Freud said to George Sylvester Viereck [1884–1962] one evening in his life, in an undeniable conversation: "I speak German and I live in a German cultural milieu. I have felt myself intellectually identified as a German for such a long time until I observed the rise of anti-Semitism in Germany and Austria. **Since then, I prefer feeling like a Jew**" [emphasis added by Sadger].

91

Let us recapitulate once more the main points: "I was born a Jew and have remained a Jew. Without much regret, I gave up the community of people the Germans denied me. Since anti-Semitism has gained the upper hand in Germany and Austria, it has made me feel like a Jew." We will have to carefully check to what extent this consciously stated view of life corresponds with the Professor's unconscious views. But first allow me to make a short historical digression.

When the revolutions of the year 1848 in the civilized countries proclaimed complete equality for all peoples, including the Jews, which the later liberal constitutions would adopt in their national basic laws, most of our comrades took the promise of equality seriously. They imagined that the golden age had come, that they were actually people like others, possessing the same duties and just as important, the same rights as Christians. And for this reason, now the most advanced among us, without further ado, were henceforth ready to no longer feel like Jews, but only like Germans, French, Swiss, etc. possessing a mosaic of beliefs. They confirmed this plan then and there through the act of placing their best strengths at the service of their respective fatherlands. But then, however, they had a sad experience. From year to year, it became more clear that full equality of all men without regard to nationality and belief existed only on uncaring paper and even the most "liberal" Christians did not go so far as to see the

Jews as members of the general community or to grant them equal rights in practice. Just a few months ago, the above-mentioned Swiss critic and poet C. A. Loosli in *The Terrible Jews* made the following statement: "In all states, one has begun to recognize the human and citizen's rights of Jews and to see them as equal under public law to the remaining citizens. But this was only the first step. The second step would have had to consist of also recognizing Jews as having equal rights socially. This would have reached a peak with the breaking up of the intellectual ghettoes. But no people now, with perhaps the exception of the English, have dared to take this step." And we may boldly add, according to communications from experts: not even the English!

One of Freud's stories in *The Interpretation of Dreams* teaches us just how subjugated the position of the Jews was before 1848:

> "I may have been ten or twelve years old, when my father began to take me with him on his walks and reveal to me in his talk his views upon things in the world we live in. Thus it was, on one such occasion, that he told me a story to show me how much better things were now than they had been in his days. 'When I was a young man,' he said, 'I went for a walk one Saturday in the streets of your birthplace; I was well dressed, and had a new fur cap on my head. A Christian

came up to me and with a single blow knocked off my cap into the mud and shouted: "Jew! get off the pavement!"' 'And what did you do?' I asked. 'I went into the roadway and picked up my cap,' was his quiet reply. This struck me as unheroic conduct on the part of the big, strong man who was holding the little boy by the hand. I contrasted this situation with another which fitted my feelings better: the scene in which Hannibal's father, Hamilcar Barca, made his boy swear before the household altar to take vengeance on the Romans. Ever since that time Hannibal had had a place in my fantasies. . . . Hannibal had been the favorite hero of my later school days. Like so many boys of that age, I had sympathized in the Punic Wars not with the Romans but with the Carthaginians. And when in the higher classes I began to understand for the first time what it meant to belong to an alien race, and anti-Semitic feelings among the other boys warned me that I must take up a definite position, the figure of the Semitic general rose still higher in my esteem. To my youthful mind Hannibal and Rome symbolized the conflict between the tenacity of Jewry and the organization of the Catholic church. And the increasing importance of the effects of the anti-Semitic movement upon our emotional life helped to fix the thoughts and feelings of those early days."

One would think that this early experience of his father—whom the son loved and idolized his entire life and whose death, according to the introduction of *The Interpretation of Dreams* was described as the most important event in his life—would have had a determinative effect on Freud's relationship to Judaism. Especially since the Zionist movement, in reaction to the ever stronger increasing anti-Semitism, continued to recruit further—even among Freud's close family. Did not Heine put these words into the mouth of his stag Hyacinth: "Judaism is not a religion at all, but bad luck!" Then the national-Jewish movement emphasized: "Being a Jew is not solely a matter of belief; it means, above all, solidarity with his people." "Zionism," as defined by [Theodor] Herzl [1860–1904], means "to return to Judaism before returning to the land of the Jews." With this program, he won the hearts of the Jewish intellectuals, and above all, the hearts of the entire Jewish youth.

Intellectuals are not very concerned with religion alone. Most of the intellectually advanced of any denomination are at best idle with respect to matters of belief and in their hearts are basically irreligious. This may hold for Jews with their sharply critical minds, perhaps in even greater numbers than for believers of other faiths. Thus the majority of them felt completely deracinated by Herzl's proposal as soon as they were no longer able to believe. There remained for them hardly options left other than to assimilate, to become as indistinguishable as possible from their Christian surroundings, even if it meant being baptized. However, such attempts to warm up to the Christians did not please the latter, but instead, as daily experience taught, mostly made the Jews the object of contempt. So the best of them were beaten back to Judaism by their enemies. Here Zionism had brought about change. From the perpetually frightened, assimilated Jew was created an upstanding group-conscious Jew, someone to whom, even the reluctant enemy, acting against its will, could not deny respect.

How did Freud, who had to experience the whole development of anti-Semitism in his own life, who encountered a double resistance against his teachings, because he was besides everything else a Jew, react to the endeavors of his people? If one reads the introductory words of this chapter, so one might believe that Freud had stood with his own people, through all times, ever since he noticed the rise of anti-Semitism. Unfortunately because my memory reaches back more than thirty years, I have much to report that is not in accord with that assumption. From the beginning, Jews formed the core group of the psychoanalytic community, certainly a good 95 percent in the first decade and a half. When later a larger number of Christians joined, they either moved away from Jewish teachings like the Swiss group under C. G. Jung or they did not accomplish anything significant. I cannot believe it was just the rarity of Christian disciples that induced Freud to make every single one of them his most special favorite. Yet the fact is that one such Christian follower was liked far more than ten of his Jewish ones. Each of them from the outset was in the master's good graces even if he was just one of the completely common crowd, even, indeed, if he was inferior. Even intellectual inferiority did not stop the Professor from personally asking him to join the innermost circle. In another case, Freud defended to the utmost one of his Christian disciples against whom serious accusations had rightly been made, and he surprisingly extolled a female student for her "beautiful name." Finally, in a fourth case, a student had made a minimal discovery, of practically no importance and this became an occasion to celebrate as a singular enrichment of *The Interpretation of Dreams,* while the work of a Jewish colleague who had nearly uncovered all of dream symbolism before Freud was not mentioned, or at best in an admonishing aside.

Basically, Freud saw in every Jew who unfailingly stood with his people something that went against his German national consciousness even though it was precisely because of his Jewishness that the German scientific establishment had shunned him. As amiable, charming, and appreciative as the Professor was towards the most insignificant Christian, he could be surly towards his able Jewish colleagues. If he did not wish a Jewish student well—and how readily this was the case!—he would find fault with the tiniest grammatical error or he would in the conversation "praise" the student's diligence by which he meant to say: You have read a great deal but what you are lacking is simply your own ideas. Most characteristic, however, was his relationship to the favorite of the gods, C. G. Jung.

I have already in earlier chapters detailed how he showered Jung with credit, praised him for discoveries which he himself had made, and finally at the Nuremberg congress, without further ado, he was ready to give away his whole young discipline to the Christian clinic. Here I must enlarge upon my previous report. While the Viennese students were stormily objecting to such suicide, and were discussing their very next steps in a side-room, the Professor appeared, uninvited, among them, and spoke with fierce agitation: "You are for the most part Jews and for that reason you are not suited to make friends for the new teachings. **Jews must resign themselves to being cultural dung. I must find a connection to the academy!**" [emphasis added by Sadger]. He, of course, never achieved the hoped-for connection to the Christian scientific establishment and such a connection would still not have happened even if the Christianization of psychoanalysis had not failed due to the objections of the Viennese students. Yes, I even dare to make the following claim: had Freud died two decades earlier, then he himself and his entire teachings in spite of all his enormous genius, would have become nothing more than mere cultural dung for the Christian scientific establishment and its representatives. Some sort of privy councilor or unknown public health officer would then have again revived psychoanalysis—obviously in a suitably proper recast form—and at most named Freud as one of its pioneers.

After all of this, I need to strongly emphasize: It is not the case, as Freud maintained, that he had always felt like a Jew. He would have liked best to have been a German and was only condemned to go back to despised Judaism very much against his will. He was, unfortunately, not able, despite all his efforts, to shed his Judaism and simply be a German. So finally he remained a Jew, though not out of loyalty to his hereditary people. Since the Christians did not want anything to do with him and his teachings, there was simply no other path open. Particularly with respect to things related to Judaism Freud's character did not stand the test of time.

If we make a comparison with two other Jewish geniuses, [Josef] Popper-Lynkeus [1838–1921] and Albert Einstein [1879–1955], this could teach us how little there is to praise about Freud's relationship to Judaism. Lynkeus, the greatest ethical genius since Baruch Spinoza [1632–1677], made much harsher judgments about all positive religions than did Freud. Yet at the end of his life, afflicted with serious illness, unable to work, he bequeathed the only thing that he still had left, his large library, to the Jewish National Library in Jerusalem. And Albert Einstein, the genius of physics, refused all invitations from money-laden snobbish America: he was too busy with his scientific work. However, when [Chaim] Weizman [1874–1952] developed his great advertising campaign for Palestine and cabled him: "Come, the Jewish people need you!" Einstein left all his scientific work behind and came to help his hard-pressed people. Freud, on the other hand, the third genius, was content to "remain a Jew," that is, he had not allowed himself to be baptized. But he was never an upstanding, consciously-aware Jew to the very end. I must unfortunately acknowledge that the human in Freud was never as great as his scientific genius!

No chapter of this little book was as hard for me to write as this one, but I promised to show the whole Freud, not just the genius, but also the fallible human. And thus, with Ammonius, I want to cry out: "Amicus Plato, sed magis amica veritas" [Plato is dear to me, but dearer still is truth, from Aristotle, *Nichomachean Ethics* I, 4, 1096a 16].

Freud and Lay Analysis

"And now there is a new parlor-game to play, psychoanalysis! One can turn this way and that, but in the end, sex is always the answer which is why it is so popular. The young
people are incredibly serious when they play it and believe
that God has shown them something exalted and erudite.
A great number of foreign words are also included so that
men can take it very seriously: instead of sex one says libido.

"Men are frightfully stupid! I come more and more to
that conclusion. They let themselves be entrapped by a
few learned phrases. As if one didn't already know all this
without such hocus pocus! But with hocus pocus, they can
all have a clear conscience. And libido sounds so refined."

Bruno Kestner, *Das Kussbuch*

The motto which I have placed above these lines shows
both the popularity as well as the little involuntary de-
tour psychoanalysis has taken in the last few years.
During the first terrible years after the war, the new
discipline did not move from the academy into wider

circles. Rather it was imported to the masses like a sport from England and America, and as a result it was mainly reduced to daily, social, and coffeehouse chatter. This growing popular interest was welcome when compared to the decade-long rejection by the academy. This interest, furthermore, lay along the path of legitimate development such that henceforth many scholars began to educate themselves about the new psychology of the unconscious and its dependence upon limited drives. Finally, it could no longer be denied that this spread of psychoanalysis proved to be an incredible stimulus among different disciplines. Only it was necessary that psychoanalysis not become degraded as a plaything for idle hours and even less as a little cloak for sultry sensuality. Practically speaking, it was worst of all that untrained doctors turned towards the new methods of treatment and in recent years even amateurs and bloody laymen.

How great the danger was can be proven by the fact that already in 1910, Freud had to take a position against "wild psychoanalysts." Such was his term for those doctors who, without really making themselves familiar with the new science, singled out just one, not even essential, point and on the basis of that gave wrong and even offensive advice. It is worth noticing and keeping in mind that Freud at that time as yet for all the years before and even for a long time afterwards wanted nothing to do with lay analysis—in contrast with his current stance. The few non-doctors who belonged at that time to the Viennese Psychoanalytic Society applied their experiences with the new discipline exclusively to their field of specialization, without actively trying to heal the mentally ill. And even the house factotum, Otto Rank was only permitted in those days to examine legendary and poetic material, and questions concerning the philosophy of religion and dreams. (In "On the History of the Psychoanalytic Movement," 1914, Freud says of Rank, "We induced him to go through the Gymnasium, and the university, and to devote himself to the non-medical application of psychoanalysis." This last also holds for Reik's beginnings.) Freud's advocacy of lay analysis to cure the ill began much later. The whole issue only became acute when the institutionalization of psychoanalytic practice, under the influence of foreign countries, began to become a profitable business.

Before I go into the question of lay analysis by outlining its pros and cons, it seems to me to be useful to deal with a few preliminary questions. Why is it that some doctors support lay analysis while others—they are the majority—are most strongly opposed? And why did Freud advocate it with such vehemence in the last few years? I don't believe a conclusive answer can be given without at least considering the historical development of the personage of the master.

In earlier chapters, I have already outlined with what unprecedented scorn, mockery, and slander Freud was subjected to over the decades. And to be sure, this happened chiefly on the part of the Viennese doctors, and especially from both those aspiring to be psychiatrists and those who were already established practitioners. It is literally true what Freud already in 1914 in "On the History of the Psychoanalytic Movement" explained:

> "In no other place is the hostile indifference of the learned and educated section of the population so evident to the analyst as in Vienna."

In 1926, in "The Question of Lay Analysis," he continued:

> "Doctors have no historical claim to the sole possession of psychoanalysis. On the contrary, until recently they have met it with everything possible that could damage it; from the shallowest ridicule to the gravest calumny."

And finally in 1927 in his "Postscript," he remembered,

> "the unfriendliness and indeed the animosity with which the medical profession treated analysis from the very first. That would seem to imply that it can have no claims over analysis today. And though I do not accept that implication, I

still feel some doubts as to whether the present wooing of psychoanalysis by the doctors is based, from the point of view of the libido theory, upon the first or upon the second of Abraham's sub-stages—whether they wish to take possession of their object for the purpose of destroying or of preserving it."

Now one must bear in mind that Sigmund Freud was always an extreme hater. That he was always able to hate by far more than he could love is connected to his strong sadistic disposition. (How little a judge of human nature can analyze himself seems strange, but is indicated when Freud in his above-mentioned "Postscript" makes the following statement: "My innate sadistic disposition was not a very strong one." The exact opposite is true, especially if one does not necessarily think of sadism in terms of the bloody deeds of the Marquis de Sade.) Now just imagine a sadist who has the ability to destroy his enemies but who at the same time is forced to remain silent in order that the new teachings associated with him will be considered. Then one can comprehend how such repression had to intensify into a lifelong hatred. (In "The Question of Lay Analysis," Freud lets the "Impartial Person" say to him, "I formed the impression that you are dominated by a hostility against the medical profession to the historical explanation of which you yourself have pointed the way.") No wonder, then, that Freud saw doctors as malevolent opponents, especially the narrow professional local colleagues in psychiatry. And unfortunately, one has to acknowledge objectively: not entirely without reason! It is humanly understandable that Freud would have felt himself more drawn toward laymen who, owing to their deficient knowledge, would be afraid to contradict him. They were unconditional supporters of their lord and master to a far greater extent than any doctor.

In comparison with this particularly decisive motivation for hatred against doctors, especially the Viennese, all other factors recede. But I will enumerate them very briefly. It was a gracious act of humanity that Freud wanted to take care of his favorite student Rank and that he allowed him to study, though not at the medical school. By directing rich English and French patients to Rank, he thus was able to take care of him, which he later continued to do with Dr. Reik as well. Finally, one can also well understand that he, as a father, was eager to take the trouble to secure the future of his daughter Anna.

Freud's above-mentioned hostility towards doctors is also betrayed in the supposed motivations for their resistance that he wanted to attribute to them in his "The Question of Lay Analysis." It seems to me worthwhile to mention how little Freud's sharp mind understood his own actions and how little he examined the reasons for his partisanship, never advising a neutral position. And it is significant that the conversion was not successful, clearly because the reasons brought forward to the high judicial official, "a man with a friendly attitude and a mind of unusual integrity" was not convinced. (Freud confirmed this himself in his "Postscript.")

But now to turn to the supposed reasons of the doctors, including Freud's own medical students and colleagues: "I think," the master said, "It must be the power of professional feeling. To impute motives of competition to them would be not only to accuse them of basic sentiments but also to attribute a strange shortsightedness to them." Practical considerations also mean nothing to him. If difficulties concerning differential diagnoses arose, these would occur no less among medical graduates who sometimes had to send their patients to a colleague because they were not allowed to physically examine them. That the patient might have less trust in a lay analyst than in a doctor of medicine is refuted by the fact that those non-doctors that practice analysis today are "not any chance collection of riffraff, but people of academic education, doctors of philosophy, educators, together with a few women of great experience in life and outstanding personality." The demands of medical knowledge grow from year to year. To expect doctors to become familiar with the mental side of illness would require a lengthening of student years, "a waste of energy for which, in these difficult times, no economic justification can be found."

Freud imagines as a preparatory institution for psychoanalysts a college that would, alongside depth psychology, teach:

"an introduction to biology, as much as possible of the science of sexual life, and familiarity with the symptomatology of psychiatry."

Furthermore, a series of "branches of knowledge"

"which are remote from medicine and the doctor does not come across in his practice: the history of civilization, mythology, the psychology of religion and the science of literature. Unless he is well at home with these subjects, an analyst can make nothing of a large amount of his material. By way of compensation, the great mass of what is taught in medical schools is of no use to him for his purposes. A knowledge of the anatomy of tarsal bones, of the constitution of hydrocarbons, of the course of cranial nerves, a grasp of all that medicine has brought to light on bacilli as exciting causes of disease and the means of combating them, on serum reactions and on neoplasms— all this knowledge, which is undoubtedly of the highest value in itself, is nevertheless of no consequence to him; it does not concern him; it neither helps him directly to understand a neurosis and to cure it nor does it contribute to a sharpening of those intellectual capacities on which his occupation makes the greatest demands."

Freud then refers further to how incredibly useful psychoanalysis could be for the humanities, if its representatives first underwent such an analysis themselves in order then to be able

"to apply its methods and angles of approach to their own materials. . . . To carry out these analyses a number of analysts will be needed, for whom any medical knowledge will have particularly little importance. But these 'teaching analysts'—let us call them—will require to have had a particularly careful education. If this is not to be stunted, they must be given an opportunity of collecting experience from instructive and informative cases; and since healthy people who also lack the motive of curiosity do not present themselves for analysis, it is once more only upon neurotics that it will be possible for the teaching analysts—under careful supervision—to be educated for their subsequent non-medical activity."

But why exclusively lay people who would first have to be educated, and who would have to have a proper training analysis which is still very rare, is not explained. Why not choose already previously psychoanalytically trained doctors? Here the logic makes little sense. Because one needs several training analyses, lay people must be trained. And if one wants to train lay people, one must allow them to treat the ill. Quod erat demonstrandum! This kind of proof reminds me a little bit of the earlier teaching institutions for blind adults. They were trained for several vocations. They learn, for example, how to make brushes and weave baskets. They can furthermore become piano tuners— and finally even teachers at institutions for the blind.

Let us follow Freud's argument further, above all with regard to the future college. We have been told what sorts of medical knowledge a proper psychoanalyst doesn't need, and what, on the other hand, he lacks. Freud was especially taken with the seven tarsal bones and the constitution of hydrocarbons. Now I know of no case in which a student was tripped up by precisely those tarsal bones during a difficult examination, and the knowledge of hydrocarbons that is required of young medical students is not nearly as detailed as that of someone who is a chemist by profession. Such examination items might now and then be annoying but certainly not life-threatening. And it is not otherwise with serum reactions and neoplasms.

On the other hand, what all does one have to learn at the future college for psychoanalysis? In addition to depth psychology, "an introduction to biology, as much as possible of the science of sexual life, familiarity with the symptomatology of psychiatry, and further, the history of civilization, mythology, the psychology of religion, and the science of literature." (In his "Postscript," Freud expands this: "A scheme of training for analysts has still to be created. It must include elements from the mental sciences, from psychology, the history of civilization and sociology, as well as from anatomy, biology and the study of evolution.") Let us consider the last-named four disciplines with which usually a doctor could at best only occasionally occupy himself out of personal interest, and certainly not focusing on more than one discipline. Any single one of these four branches of knowledge would require a whole lifetime, or, should we say more modestly, many years of a life if one were to undertake it in earnest and not as a mere bloody dilettante—certainly far more time than to study tarsal bones together with serum reactions. But, however, add to these the first four named medical or half-medical subjects. How will one teach the listeners "as much as possible about the science of sexual life" without also covering normal and pathological anatomy and physiology, and not just of the sexual organs but the whole nervous, muscular and vascular system, and one can hardly ignore also the other glands of the body and that means endocrinology (the study of inner secretion, the secretions of the so-called blood glands). And the "symptomatology of psychiatry" is hard enough to remember without frequent visits to a mental institution and without at least a more detailed study of the brain.

I have two kinds of objections to Freud's proposals: They expand the teaching plan of psychoanalysis improperly in one direction and let it contract improperly in the other. One could, for example, ask why are only just those four humanities emphasized, though to be sure, in the "Postscript" it was expanded to include sociological materials just as it was expanded in the medical direction to include anatomy and the study of evolution. It would be hard to believe that these four disciplines were picked out because doctors of philosophy Rank and Reik had just worked in them. After all, the yearly runs of *Imago* and the *Zeitschrift für psychoanalytische Pädagogik* conclusively show how art and art history, anthropology, linguistics, and above all, childhood education have already contributed a great deal, not to mention other sources. If one absorbs all this into the teaching plan for the future college, then it will grow into an unlimited philosophical department with a smaller medical appendage. Then, however, one will have an amount of material to learn so vast that no individual would be able to learn it in one lifetime. I'm afraid that a listener in such a college would stand, in terms of basic knowledge, barely higher than an educated lay person, or above a nurse as far as medical knowledge is concerned.

When Freud in his "Postscript," asks of analysts that they

"should overcome the one-sidedness that is fostered by instruction in medical schools and that they should resist the temptation to flirt with endocrinology and the autonomic nervous system, when what is needed is an apprehension of psychological facts with the help of a framework of psychological concepts"

then I must respond: Those doctors who are now practicing psychoanalysis are far from being one-sided. They neither have the time nor the will to indulge in such peripheral studies. Even the youngest, most knowledge-hungry colleagues are content with the two years spent in a psychiatric clinic, the preliminary study required in order to familiarize themselves with nervous and mental diseases. I cannot name a single individual who has intensely focused on inner secretions or the autonomic nervous system, or who would have let his psychoanalytic technique be influenced by such things.

Freud agreed that

"the great principles of pathology—the theories of inflammation, suppuration, necrosis, and of the metabolism of the bodily organs—still retain their importance"

for dentists who represent a particular specialization but who in Austria are required to be doctores universae medicinae. But there is, however, also an "organic component" with psychoneuroses, that is surely of decisive importance during interaction. On a theoretical level, we can follow this interaction more clearly by observing the master himself. I don't think that any dentist is influenced by "the great principles" more than Freud is by endocrinology. Did he not do more than merely "flirt" with endocrinology in the fourth edition of his "Three Essays on the Theory of Sexuality" by giving up his earlier sexual toxicity theory in favor of a newer inner secretion one? Further: in the "Postscript" he tells us that he spent a lot of time studying zoology, chemistry and histology, without these studies, which were hardly less superfluous for an understanding of psychoanalysis than the study of tarsal bones, preventing him from becoming Freud. Yes, perhaps one might risk claiming that it was precisely the critical influence of [Ernst] Brücke [1819–1892] "the greatest authority that ever influenced him" and his exactitude in psychological methods that were decisive for Freud's having such a perceptive attitude towards the problems of psychoanalysis. Finally, I want to stress that recently even sensible doctors such as Eugen Bleuler have been enthusiastically advocating the psychological permeation of all medicine.

Since the master has merely told us over and over what the doctors neglected and have not done, we want for once to put forth a short counter-claim. What have these highly praised lay people accomplished for psychoanalysis up to now? Certainly, they have applied to

the humanities what Freud and his doctor collaborators discovered and everyone mastering a special area
benefited greatly from the purely medical discoveries.
But, however, how do things look in reverse? Has any
lay person discovered any psychoanalytic truth that has
enriched our medical activity or our knowledge, a truth
that did not purely and simply derive from or confirm
what Freud in his genius had already previously taught
us? Even if the master secretly gave them his ideas
which was not a rare occurrence, a knowledgeable person would notice in an instant this graft of his great intuition. Even where lay persons do have a unique place,
in child analysis, the decisive model in all of the roots of
its methodology and understanding came from the
interpretation and treatment of the phobia of Little
Hans. If we are to find lay analysts indispensable, then
one must also find their achievements indispensable or
creative. But to this day, such proof has not yet materialized and probably never will. (Ernst [sic] Jones who is
usually an opponent of lay analysis does argue in its
favor by mentioning Hans [sic] Sachs "provided contributions to many technical questions" and "the most
striking example of symbolism. In a whole series of examples, the study of folklore and of comparative religion, etc., has revealed to us the significance and understanding of continually recurring symbols that until
then had remained unknown to us in our clinical
work." To this we can only respond that Hans Sachs'

technical innovations can hardly be discovered with a naked eye, and that for an understanding of symbolism, we have nothing to thank the lay people for, but rather Dr. Stekel who in his *Conditions of Nervous Anxiety and Their Treatment* [1908] and later *The Language of Dreams* [1911] before anyone taught us to understand dreams. Even Freud himself in the first edition of his *Interpretation of Dreams* did not yet know this symbolism. Now I know very well that Stekel is outlawed in psychoanalytic circles and also that no one can ascribe to me a particular fondness or even a weakness for him. But there remains one law of scientific decorum and that is to acknowledge merit, even that of opponents. And therefore I am obliged to say: It was not lay people who opened up for us the understanding of symbolism, but Wilhelm Stekel on the basis of his medical psychoanalyses!)

One can thus summarize something like this: The collaboration of lay people has until now merely confirmed what was discovered by doctors, mostly by Freud, and has never contributed anything really new or therapeutically exceptional. The psychoanalytic healing method and the new psychology created by it can exist without difficulty without drawing upon lay activity of any kind. If we leave aside child analysis, therapy would not suffer the slightest loss without lay analysis. On the other hand, the humanities would be deprived of an important possible means of insight if they ignored psychoanalytic findings. It is, however, of no consequence whether these findings are transmitted to them by doctors or by specialists who were psychoanalytically trained.

Freud is constantly tormented by the fear that psychoanalysis will become "swallowed up" by medicine which is so hostile to it. I cannot share this concern at all especially because its technique is so hard to learn. The old privy councilors will certainly not do it, and even the Assistants in psychiatry have up until now not had much to do with psychoanalysis. On the other hand, it is again not understandable why a lay person who wished to apply psychoanalytic insights to anthropology or linguistics would first need to devote years of work learning all the tricks of the technique. It would suffice if each lay person let himself be analyzed, and that he mastered the psychoanalytic literature.

Freud's book *The Question of Lay Analysis* consists of two parts: a first part which in its brilliant and lucid expression recalls the best times of the master, and a second, later part, whose arguments are extremely vulnerable.

I want to add the following to all that I have already said: The critical question seems to me to be: Is the practice of the psychoanalytic treatment of neurotics a medical activity or not? I believe there can be no doubt at all about the answer. And if the question needs to be answered with an emphatic yes, then the treatment necessarily should be reserved for medical psychoanalysts. There is also, however, as practice teaches, important medical hesitations about lay analysis. It is readily pointed out that a medical investigation always comes first and, on the other hand, that doctors of medicine now and then are forced to demand help from their colleagues. Here, however, lies the essential difference between lay and medical treatment.

As a practical matter, the confusion between hysteria and schizophrenia has proven to be the most significant and dangerous mistake. It goes without saying that even a doctor who is himself both neurologist and psychiatrist at the beginning of a differential diagnosis cannot always decide with certainty. Then when he begins an analysis, it is mostly in the first hours that he can diagnose the probable psychosis or at the very least can make a very strong guess and then take appropriate measures. Experience teaches that it is just at this point that the lay analyst is easily surprised by the unexpected outbreak of schizophrenia, which then puts all of psychoanalysis in a bad light.

Now, however, to the much more frequent cases of conversion hysteria and anxiety. We know that during the course of being treated for a host of symptoms that occur, the patient without exception always attributes them to some kind of physical cause or severe organic affect. And, to be sure, the outbreak of nervous symptoms and the constant anxiety associated with them are not always something occasional, but rather occur repeatedly and so often that they become the center of all complaints. Here the lay analyst now gets into a difficult situation that a doctor hardly encounters. If he is conscientious, then he must send the patient to a doctor for every single complaint which, the more often this is repeated, will hardly increase the trust of the patient in the analyst. Or if he is less conscientious, however, and says to himself, "Oh, the patient is probably just being hysterical again!" then it is quite possible that he will overlook an organic affect or a psychosis with all the consequences that arise from this.

I hope I am not committing an act of indiscretion if I cite a blatant example. Dr. [Hermine] Hug-Helmut [1871–1924], who was perhaps the most qualified child analyst, often confessed to me her reflections, her doubts whether or not a lack of medical education might cause her to overlook or not recognize something. She questioned me with every individual case to get medical advice. Since we often collaborated in joint scientific work, she had ample opportunity to seek reassurance. But now what about the other lay analysts? Not everyone has "the university at home" as Anna Freud does. In most cases, lay analysts will either be too conscientious or not sufficiently conscientious with all of the above-mentioned consequences. In contrast, the medical psychoanalyst who has had not just neurological-psychiatric training, but general medical training will be able to decide for himself with certainty from the type of complaint presented what measures to take and only in the rarest of cases, or if the patient himself requests it, will he have to refer the patient to a specialist. He will, however, also be able to say to the patient, "I am referring you because you are urgently pressing me to do so, but I am telling you that it is unnecessary, that there is nothing physically wrong with you and that you are throwing your money out the window."

Although Freud has faith that the general public will know itself how to decide when to turn to a doctor or to a lay analyst, everyday experience speaks against this. Today, "Höllerhansl" (a southern Austrian quack who ascertains all illnesses from urine samples and cures them with herbs) has a far greater crowd of patients and is busier that the most experienced, ablest internists. And it is of no use to have a later rational reflection after a patient has once been damaged by a less conscientious lay analyst. Such a patient might then, having become wiser, not turn towards a medical analyst, but instead simply throw the whole entire healing method overboard. Probably he would go to our competitors. But certainly he would complain a lot, taking care to give the widest dissemination of our failures.

We have heard above which wonderful qualities Freud has ascribed to lay analysts. They are not "any chance collection of riffraff, but people of academic education, doctors of philosophy, educationists, together with a few women of great experience in life and outstanding personality." This might have been the case as long as one could count the "healing" lay analysts on the fingers of one hand. But this is no longer generally true and from year to year will become even less true as further cohorts of lay analysts turn towards treatment of the ill. Most English, Americans and Dutch have sufficiently recognized this while among most Austrian and German doctors, Freud, through the sheer power of his personality—not his argument—has silenced tentative hesitations. When Freud boasted in his "Postscript," that "many colleagues have reduced their extreme *parti pris* and that the majority has accepted his view," the truth is that at least 90 percent of the psychoanalytic medical community would have rejected treatment by lay analysts had not Freud and a few blind followers been at work. There were, however, two kinds of reasons for the famous "reduction" of partiality: First of all, backbone and strength of character are not very widespread in the world and doctors constitute no great exception, and secondly, no one in the least among the medical analysts wanted to stand up against Freud, the venerated one. They preferred to be persuaded that the lay analysts were "secular caretakers of souls," the enticing bait that Freud threw at them. But what impels so many lay persons without medical and psychiatric training among other omissions in training to treat neurotics is hardly the need to be "secular caretakers of souls" nor a desire to gain knowledge or understanding, but rather in most cases doubtless the prospect of a prosperous business. Lay analysis promises to become a lucrative living. Take away from them the possibility of well-paid hours and let them work without any compensation and the grand enthusiasm for the secular caretaking of souls would quickly die down.

If you will permit me, I will conclude this section with the same sentences that I have already used once in the discussion of lay analysis: "I firmly believe that patients should be treated exclusively by doctors and that any lay analysis should be avoided by them. The only exception I would allow is the educational healing of children and adolescents. Here it is a matter of a sense of how a child is raised, a sense that doctors and even pediatricians possess only in the rarest cases, and only secondarily of medical knowledge. And besides, every male doctor runs the risk to begin with of being perceived as a father figure from whom the adolescent fears the threat of castration, a threat which for a mother or mother-imago is much less or doesn't exist at all. But the adult neurotic absolutely requires a doctor. It may indeed be very useful for doctors of philosophy and other lay persons to do their utmost to familiarize themselves with the results of psychoanalysis to help them in their different disciplines to achieve better comprehension and to know how to bring this knowledge to those proper experts who do not have this training. Lay persons can here be an extraordinary blessing, each for his own special discipline. Indeed, in their hands, psychoanalysis can have an even more stimulating effect than evolutionary theory, Darwinism, had decades ago. But from the treatment of adult neurotics who require purely psychoanalytic general medical knowledge together with special neurological-psychiatric training, lay persons should absolutely keep far away—even if they are doctors of philosophy."

From the Last Years of Freud's Life

It was in the fall of the year 1923 when I heard the terrible news that Freud had become ill due to a malignant growth on the upper jaw that then had been operated on. The cancer had returned and spread which had made a second operation necessary. The doctors had given the patient at most just one year to live. The mood of the disciples was deeply depressed. And even when Freud appeared again in the year 1924 to speak to the Society, no one could really be happy about this sign of life. The impression made by the Professor's speech was simply horrible. Already the pale, deeply sunken face had an extremely sad look. And when one heard what had formerly been so melodious a voice sound distressed, one could tell by the bad sound how affected his speech was. Everyone looked down, embarrassed, their eyes lowered. Nevertheless, what Freud said still remained at the same high level as before, only one had to first, with some difficulty, get used to the new tonality. We could not hide this reaction from the Professor and he did not appear again thereafter until the obsequies for Karl Abraham in the year 1926 drew him back to the Society one last time for a very brief moment.

Also what the most intimate members of the group reported did not sound very encouraging. They described the deep depression of the Professor during the first months: "I am a dead man, Don't count on me any more !" One has to keep in mind that the death complex had always been very strong in Freud. I remember, for example, the psychoanalytic congress in Nuremberg. On the afternoon before, Freud himself set out on a walk, followed by a group of his disciples. And to what place did his path lead? To the cemetery, far beyond the city, although he had no precious grave to visit. So he was always drawn to the dead. And he even took an immediate interest in people who had been entirely unsympathetic to him as soon as he heard of their death and he never forgot to send his condolences. It always remained that the surest way to attract Freud's attention was to lie down and die.

The Professor wrote one of his best essays when the World War with its massacres was at its height: "Thoughts for the Times on War and Death" [1915]. I extract from it the following passages:

"Our attitude towards death was far from straightforward. To anyone who listened to us we were of course prepared to maintain that death was the necessary outcome of life, that everyone owes nature a death and must expect to pay the debt—in short, that death was natural, undeniable and unavoidable. In reality, however, we were accustomed to behave as if it were otherwise. We showed an unmistakable tendency to put death on one side, to eliminate it from life. We tried to hush it up; indeed we even have a saying: 'to think of something as though it were death!' That is, as though it were our own death, of course. It is indeed impossible to imagine our own death; and whenever we attempt to do so we can perceive that we are in fact still present as spectators. Hence the psychoanalytic school could venture on the assertion that at bottom no one believes in his own death, or, to put the same thing in another way, that in the unconscious everyone of us is convinced of his own immortality.

"When another person dies, we are always deeply affected, and it is as though we were badly shaken in our expectations. Our habit is to lay stress on the fortuitous causation of the death—accident, disease, infection, advanced age; in this way we betray an effort to reduce death from a necessity to a chance event . . . Towards the actual person who has died we adopt a special attitude—something almost like admiration for someone who has accomplished a very difficult task."

Finally someone close to us dies, and then

"Our hopes, our desires and our pleasures lie in the grave with him, we will not be consoled, we will not fill the lost one's place. We behave as if we were a kind of Asra, **who die when those they love die**." [emphasis added by Sadger]

If we disregard the experiences of war, then

"the question arises. . . . Should we not confess that in our civilized attitude towards death we are once again living psychologically beyond our means, and should we not rather turn back and recognize the truth? Would it not be better to give death the place in reality and in our thoughts which is its due, and to give a little more prominence to the unconscious attitude towards death which we have hitherto so carefully suppressed? . . . The old saying: *Si vis pacem, para bellum.* 'If you want to preserve peace, arm for war' could be changed in keeping with the times to: *Si vis vitam, para mortem.* 'If you want to endure life, prepare yourself for death.'"

Freud based the remainder of his life on this formula, bravely preparing himself for death by using to advantage his ability whenever possible in the service of his teachings. Of course, he knew well enough that his days were numbered, but like Heine, he showed in suffering all his greatness of character. If he had initially withdrawn from all activity during the first moments of shock, so he now tried to take over in person the leadership of the Viennese Psychoanalytic Society and when this attempt failed, he directed it at the very least out of his own home as he did the agenda of the International Association. Also as a teacher, he contributed whatever he still had to contribute. Nothing more in the way of groundbreaking—that his illness would not permit—but he certainly perfected and finalized older thoughts, such as "The Passing of the Oedipus Complex" [1924], "The Economic Problem in Masochism" [1924], "Some Psychological Consequences of the Anatomical Distinction between the Sexes" [1925], "Humour" [1928], "Fetishism" [1927], as well as larger works such as *Inhibitions, Symptoms, and Anxiety* [1926] and *The Question of Lay Analysis* [1926]. And finally, *The Future of an Illusion* [1927]. All of these works, written in a classic popular style, developed the whole underlying structure of psychoanalysis.

Feeling too weak to preside over meetings on a far-away street until some time around midnight, he now returned to the beginnings of his teaching activity and invited old and new students to his own home. Once a month, they met to present their latest ideas and what was even more important for them, to hear the opinion of the master himself and to listen to his wisdom and experience. If they were lucky and he was in a good spirits, then they could imagine they had the young Freud in front of them. He had managed to make his method of teaching be even more direct than in earlier years. Back in the old days, it was the custom to first let the speaker finish followed then by the voices of the critics, the sequence of which actually determined the fate of the speaker. But now the Professor thought it would serve his cause better if he—naturally only he himself—raised objections on the spot as they occurred to him. For example, one of the younger members of the Society had come up with his own technique and wanted to convert the others to it. He believed that one must first, before going back to search for original causes and associations, merely tease out the resistance of the patient and immediately control it. Here the old practitioner balked and when the speaker began to tell how he had come upon his method, the master interrupted him: "Oh, I see. Previously you paid too little attention to resistance and then you became smarter through mistakes and now you have gone to the other extreme." Among the guests was Princess [Marie] Bonaparte of Greece [1882–1962], one of Freud's students, who was listening intently. To her the Professor now turned with a kindly smile, "I believe that one has to attack the enemy where one encounters him. What do you think about that, Princess?"

How delightfully Freud could converse when he was having one of his good evenings. He would begin to draw from his memories, weave in a joke here and a deep insight there, and enthrall the audience into deeply respectful admiration by means of the most charming manner. He would quote from his favorite poet Nestroy, for example, the following words: "It is a cross to bear for people! All the world complains about the bad weather and no one does anything about it!" Or he would vent his anger on the different garbage-movements derived from his teachings, painting a startling picture. These offshoot movements appeared to him as if dogs had jumped on a table on which a magnificent meal had been prepared. Each dog dragged off a bone from there and ran with it into another corner of the room. Now and then, he could almost be truly humorous. On those occasions, he played with things and by this means produced a new fascinating effect.

I remember one evening where the topic of neurotic actual-conflict was the subject of debate. After the initial speaker had presented her opening remarks, basically no one had anything more to say. However, to get a conversation going, a member seized upon the word "actual-conflict" and led astray by sound associations, began to talk and play around with "actual neuroses" which was eagerly picked up by the others. The battle over these new spoils of war raged back and forth for some time until finally the Professor interrupted: "This reminds me of a silly anecdote, but one that fits the occasion quite well. A candidate was supposed to be examined in zoology, but he, however, had only learned about the elephant. Unfortunately, he was asked about the hyena, and he began thus: 'The hyena is an ugly, a disgusting animal, but how handsome, on the other hand, is the elephant! There are two types of elephant: the African and the Indian.' And thus he started off and tied everything up neatly in a ball of string all that he had learned. Now permit me to say a few words on the topic." (This reminds me of another charming anecdote, one about the late neurologist, Professor Moritz Benedikt [1835–1920], who was for a long time the leader of the democratic party in Vienna. This professor was asked by a doctor to come to the bed of a patient with a hopeless spinal cord injury for a consultation. After examining the patient, Benedikt went back to the doctor and said to him, "Dear colleague, there is nothing more we can do to help the patient, but wouldn't you like to become a member of the central union of the democratic party?")

Then came a few sentences from his enormous experience that were worth more than the entire previous discussion. Again, I felt myself transported back to the classical age of psychoanalysis where one came just simply for one single illumination from the master to carry home as a life-long treasure.

It should not be kept secret here that there were days on which the master just sat there, tired and broken. This was usually shortly before the beginning of his summer holiday, a decline in the routine. Then he would speak very little, and, if need be, even breaking up the meeting somewhat early. At other times, he was at his peak, at least for a little while. However, even on his bad days, he was impressive through the combination of his personage and teachings. If, for instance, one of the students had gone too far in his lecture, and had according to his own course of development "expanded" on the Professor's teachings, then the master would refute him with a single sentence. Or if that student finally after a longer digression managed to say something with passion that Freud had already said twenty years before, only very much more clearly, he would say to the student good-naturedly and ironically: "I am sure I have read that somewhere before."

In order to prevent any legends or erroneous impressions from developing, I want to expressly state something that all those present at those last evenings would confirm, that Freud never recanted his teachings in the least. He explicitly held fast to some of his oldest views such as the cause of neurasthenia and anxiety neurosis, as well as the formation of both these types of illness. As far as individual points that he had outgrown were concerned, he corrected them himself in later publications, so no one can claim that he was unfaithful to his original opinions outside of those he corrected himself.

Here and there, Freud experienced in his homeland some small satisfaction, but not anything from the university or the government, both of which took no notice of the genius in their midst, acts of remarkable consistency. Nor did he receive the Nobel prize. One can see how things go in medicine, not just in psychiatry. One man is a genius and achieves immortality but another receives the Nobel prize. So nature compensates for the dissimilarity of their contributions. In contrast, strangely enough, the city council of Vienna, led and governed by the social democratic party, paid some attention. On his seventieth birthday, Freud was granted as a special honor, the same as an assistant chairman would have received, namely, the simple right of citizenship of the city. But, of course, the council assumed that the Professor would hardly make much use of the "benefits" associated with the honor. At the same time, however, the council turned over twenty-one official consulting positions to "Comrade" Alfred Adler. When, however, several comrades, attracted by Freud's genius, had later joined our circle, they arranged to have a not-all-that-large grassy plot given to our Society, a space the council did not know what to do with. It was not exactly ideally located, between the city jail, a future police barracks, and the "flea market" (the Viennese second-hand goods hall). In addition, instead of granting a yearly subvention for the hundreds of citizens treated free of charge, the city, in all kinds of limiting clauses and restrictions, charged an annual licensing fee. Nevertheless, it was a piece of property on which one could build a proper home for psychoanalytic research—with one's own money. (When Freud was told about the transfer of this piece of property in the Bergasse, he replied ironically: "For a mountain expedition we thus already have the naked knee.")

In the winter before last, Freud had already significantly reduced the number of meetings at his home. Partly a prevailing flu epidemic, partly a cold gave him occasion to decline all further invitations. At one of the few gatherings, he once spoke of how much life had lost its charm for him: in speaking, he was severely handicapped, eating and drinking he could enjoy only a little, and what was the worst of all, he had to almost completely give up his much beloved smoking. And then since his severe illness had so debilitated him, it made him unable to serve his discipline as he had in earlier years. He was, furthermore, occupied mainly with caring for his large family with whom he was still pleased to practice psychoanalysis for many hours daily. In a posthumous poem by Goethe, I read a verse that seemed to me to be aimed at Freud:

"The gods, the infinite ones,
Give to their favorites, everything,
All the joys, the infinite ones
All the pains, the infinite ones—everything!"

❦

In the holy city of Jerusalem sat old Ram-Bam, Rabbi Moses ben Maimon, on a high chair in the large school in front of a circle of many hundreds of students who were listening to his wisdom. (This saint's legend I related to Elise Orzeszkowa [1842–1910] including the historical error that Ram-Bam had lived and worked in Jerusalem.) And when he finished speaking, his best student, Rabbi Jehuda stood up: "One thing in the Bible I don't understand. Perhaps you could explain it to me. Who were the angels our forefather Jacob dreamed of, who climbed up on a ladder to heaven and then returned to earth [Genesis 28:12]?" Rabbi Moses thought a long time, but then the answer flowed from his lips: "These angels are great men, they are accomplished and wise, that is, they climb always higher. It becomes hard for them, but yet they manage to succeed in climbing ever higher because they possess great strength and desire. They will reach a place where they will find enlightenment and perfection. And whether they are called prophets, wise men, or men of great spirit, they are all angels that climb the ladder to God's heaven." So spoke Rabbi Moses. But Rabbi Jehuda was still not satisfied and he asked further: "Why do they go up and then come down again? If they are striving to reach the top, why don't they stay there instead of coming back down to earth? Ram-Bam then shook his white hair like the mane of a lion, "If they stayed up and never returned, they would be humans and not angels! Up above, they acquire gentleness and enlightenment and then they climb down in order to disseminate these treasures on earth. And the ground on which they disperse their seed produces better grain. From it sprouts no more discord, but peace instead, and people weep less and rejoice more. That is why they like to come back to earth, as hard as it is for them, and that is why, Rabbi Jehuda, that is why they are angels!"

That is why they are angels! Such an angel was also Sigmund Freud who sowed the seed of a new idea so that men would become happier. And the teachings which he presented for the first time in 1893 and which he devoted the whole rest of his life to always further amplifying and refining, these teachings have proven to be incredibly enlightening. Darwinism attained a similar, fruitful influence in the last century of humanity but by no means to such a large degree. Originally created as a method for curing neuroses, psychoanalysis has become, above all, the first true psychiatry for the healthy as well as for the ill human, and it has spread in many directions to solve questions, riddles, and problems against which many generations of researchers have painfully butted their heads in vain. At the present time, there is no field in the humanities that, for better or worse, does not refer to Sigmund Freud and psychoanalysis. One may find fault with many individual aspects, and to be sure, no teaching is built for eternity. There is also no doubt that if its creator had not become so ill, he himself might have modified many things. But in spite of all imperfections and incompleteness, how powerfully his new teaching has taken hold and towered over all conventional knowledge!

Ibsen's "enemy of the people" [1882], Dr. Stockmann, claims in his great speech, "A normal constituted truth lives, let us say, as a rule, seventeen or eighteen, or at most twenty years; seldom longer. But truths as aged as that are always worn frightfully thin, and nevertheless it is only then that the majority recognizes them and recommends them to the community as wholesome moral nourishment." The fate of Freudian teachings was substantially different. They took almost twice as long to develop, were not recognized by the majority, much less recommended. But for that reason, they are alive and remain as fresh as they were at their beginnings, and will be for decades, in all probability, the basis of psychiatry and the science of mankind. It is a dangerous thing about which to prophesy, but in spite of that, I will dare to make the claim that not one hundred, perhaps not fifty, years will pass after the death of Freud and posterity will place him amongst the ranks of Newton and Copernicus. What was small and mortal of him and his teachings will have disappeared without a trace. What will remain, however, is an infinite gain in the understanding of mankind.